The Jossey-Bass Health Care Series brings together the most current information and ideas in health care from the leaders in the field. Titles from the Jossey-Bass Health Care Series include these essential health care resources:

Achieving Impressive Customer Service: 7 Strategies for the Health Care Manager, Wendy Leebov, Gail Scott, Lolma Olson

Breakthrough Performance: Accelerating the Transformation of Health Care Organizations, Ellen J. Gaucher, Richard J. Coffey

Curing Health Care: New Strategies for Quality Improvement, Donald M. Berwick, A. Blanton Godfrey, Jane Roessner

Customer Service in Health Care: A Grassroots Approach to Creating a Culture of Excellence, Kristin Baird

Improving Clinical Practice: Total Quality Management and the Physician, David Blumenthal, Ann C. Scheck, Editors

Managing Patient Expectations: The Art of Finding and Keeping Loyal Patients, Susan Keane Baker

Measuring and Managing Patient Satisfaction, 2nd Edition, William Krowinski, Ph.D., Steven Steiber, Ph.D.

Profiting from Quality: Outcomes Strategies for Medical Practice, Steven Isenberg, Richard Gliklich

Provider Report Cards: A Guide for Promoting Health Care Quality to the Public, Patrice Spath, Editor

Service Savvy Health Care: One Goal at a Time, Wendy Leebov, Susan Afriat, Jeanne Presha

Total Customer Satisfaction: A Comprehensive Approach for Health Care Providers, Stephanie G. Sherman, V. Clayton Sherman

Total Quality in Healthcare: From Theory to Practice, Ellen J. Gaucher, Richard J. Coffey

Communicating with Today's Patient

Communicating with Today's Patient

Essentials to Save Time, Decrease Risk, and Increase Patient Compliance

JOANNE DESMOND and
LANNY R. COPELAND, M.D.

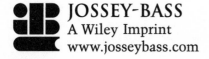
JOSSEY-BASS
A Wiley Imprint
www.josseybass.com

Published by Jossey-Bass
A Wiley Imprint
989 Market Street, San Francisco, CA 94103-1741 www.josseybass.com

Jossey-Bass books and products are available through most bookstores. To contact Jossey-Bass directly call our Customer Care Department within the U.S. at 800-956-7739, outside the U.S. at 317-572-3986 or fax 317-572-4002.

Jossey-Bass also publishes its books in a variety of electronic formats. Some content that appears in print may not be available in electronic books.

Some of the material in this book is based on work developed by David W. Merrill, Ph.D., and is copyrighted by the Cahners TRACOM Group, Denver, Colorado. The term "Social Style^{sm}" is a service mark of the Cahners TRACOM Group and is used by permission.

Library of Congress Cataloging-in-Publication Data

Desmond, Joanne, date
    Communicating with today's patient: essentials to save time, decrease risk, and increase patient compliance / Joanne Desmond and Lanny R. Copeland; foreword by Bruce Dan.
        p. cm.—(Jossey-Bass health care series)
    Includes bibliographical references and index.
    ISBN 0-7879-4797-0 (pbk. : alk. paper)
    1. Physician and patient. 2. Health counseling. 3. Patient compliance. I. Copeland, Lanny R. II. Title. III. Series.
    R727.3.D46 2000
    610.69'6—dc21
                                                                    00-010404

PB Printing   10 9 8 7 6 5 4   FIRST EDITION

CONTENTS

Foreword   ix
Bruce B. Dan, M.D.

Preface   xiii

Acknowledgments   xxi

1   Ten Reasons You Need to Read This Book   1

2   Tips to Keep New Patients and Build Your Practice   13

3   Patient Personalities and How They Affect   37
    Your Practice

4   Louder Than Words: What Your Body Language Says   71
    to Patients

5   Listening Techniques for Faster, More Accurate   95
    Diagnoses

6   Explanations Patients Can Understand   135
    and Remember

7   Communicating About Medications   165

 8   **Effectively Interacting with the Patient's Family**   187

 9   **Communicating Across Borders and Language Barriers**   203

10   **Shining Up Your Professional Image**   221

     Conclusion   237

     CME Information and Test   239

     Bibliography and References   247

     Recommended Reading   253

     Index   255

     About the Authors   263

     About Desmond Medical Communications   265

FOREWORD

It's impossible to know how many times every day poor communication occurs, in every medical office throughout the country. The number must be staggering, and the consequences even more so.

Although physicians and patients come to the examining table with the best of intentions, an impartial observer would often see physicians saying one thing and patients hearing another. Today's medical system portrays people desperately trying to relate their problems, while their doctors are clearly (or unclearly) perceiving things quite differently. Medications taken improperly. Instructions not followed. Advice not heeded. Complaints not heard. Unhappy patients, unhappy professionals, and lawsuits waiting in the wings. As the saying goes, what we have here is failure to communicate.

I've spent most of my professional life studying and writing about communication in a global nature. As senior editor of the *Journal of the American Medical Association,* I spoke to my profession about the need to communicate better; as medical editor of ABC News, Chicago, I talked to the public about how to communicate with doctors. The authors of *Communicating with Today's Patient,* Joanne Desmond and Lanny Copeland, have focused their efforts in a related communications arena: that of researching medical interactions, analyzing them, and educating individual physicians on how to practice effective one-on-one communication with their patients. In this book, they share what they have learned; perhaps most important for busy practicing clinicians, they give us insightful and useful tips on how to become more adept communicators and better doctors.

I've known Joanne for more than a decade and have watched admiringly in her physician workshops. She has the knack of grabbing physicians' attention, earning their respect, and—in a short span—changing them into adept professional communicators. I've also been fortunate to teach communication skills with her, and it's always enlightening to see workshop participants markedly improve their communications ability after learning just a few simple techniques.

When you meet a patient for the first time, do you know how to say hello most effectively? Have you ever observed or had someone else observe your body language as you talk to a patient? Have you ever written in the medical chart the color of your patient's eyes? The authors tell you why you should do so, and they offer many other clever hints as well. From tips on knocking on the door of the examining room to wrapping up the patient interview and saying goodbye, Joanne Desmond and Lanny Copeland take you through the optimal patient encounter. You'll learn how to be an empathic listener, how to talk to a patient's family, and even how to avoid the "hot buttons" that can destroy a relationship with a patient.

Does this demand more of your time in the hurry-up, managed care world of modern medicine? The authors point out that it can actually save you time, save you money, and, most important, bring back the joy of taking care of patients. These "communication pearls" result in better diagnoses, loyal and healthier patients, decreased malpractice claims, and greater professional satisfaction.

Like you, I've had the privilege over the course of my medical career of seeing and treating thousands of patients. I've seen them in office practice, in teaching institutions, and in clinical research settings. We've had conversations in private rooms in university medical centers, in U.S. Army barracks, and in open wards in Veterans Administration hospitals. What these interactions all had in common was the shared experience of working together to solve a problem.

When I entered the world of medical practice more than twenty-five years ago, clinical practice was for the most part a simple, private, one-on-one interaction with a patient. Not so in today's medical world. For many, medical practice seems to have become a daily competitive grind, aided and abetted by third-party payers, managed care organizations, and governmental bureaucracies. As a colleague of mine recently related, "Practice today is regulation, exasperation, and strangulation!" So, the question is not how we found ourselves in this miserable mess (the obvious answer, I suggest, is the fragmentation of the doctor-patient relationship), but how we get out of it.

The answers to many of the problems in medical practice today can be found, I suspect, in better patient communication. I argue that communicating well is not only a valuable clinical skill but—with today's patient—one that is critical and essential. As the authors of this book state often, if the patient-physician encounter can become a shared experience, the results are fewer complaints and greater satisfaction on both sides of the examining table.

Some people say that most communications problems in medicine are due to perception rather than reality. But when it comes to communication, perception often *is* reality. What is heartening to note is that better patient communication also results in better medical care.

If you are involved in clinical practice of medicine, you simply have to learn these techniques in communication skills. After reading this book, you'll be able to understand and use them. Read the book, and practice what the authors preach. You and your patients will be the beneficiaries.

Bruce B. Dan, M.D.
Assistant Adjunct Professor
Preventive Medicine
Vanderbilt University School of Medicine

PREFACE

Gifted with a high IQ, you probably would have been successful in many fields and in most areas of the sciences: chemistry, biology, physics. So what brought you into medicine? Helping others must have had a significant appeal for you, and you probably chose medicine partly so that you could have a direct, positive impact on people's lives.

But has that noble calling been reduced to a faint whisper or a distant sigh amid the daily crush of patients? Interacting positively with large numbers of patients can be stressful, physically and mentally, particularly with today's patients—something of a new breed.

When patients are changeable, switching from provider to provider, it can leave you discouraged, wondering what went wrong. Yet patients are often just as unhappy about switching, feeling like transients, forced to hastily bundle up their health concerns and move on each time their company's benefits or retirement plan changes.

When patients are outspoken, even demanding, about their health care, or when they seek referrals to specialists or high-tech tests to back up their self-diagnoses, it can be frustrating for you. Yet patients' voices are increasingly heard, as they are encouraged by the popular media to take an active role in their own health care.

I often hear complaints of this type from clinicians in the Desmond Medical Communications workshops. Participants report that some managed care patients come in with an almost palpable sense of entitlement: "Hey, look! I paid into this up front, so I'm entitled to my CT scan." But we also hear the complaints of patients who say they are receiving too little attention and must speak up and assert themselves to be heard or heeded.

Adding to the tension is the clock, ticking, ticking! How often are you double-booked, even triple-booked, and running behind? Time constraints compound the difficulties of communicating positively.

At times it seems like a no-win situation. If you grant patients' requests and refer them to the specialists they want or give them the tests they insist on, it can have unpleasant consequences for you. Your professional evaluation scores may suddenly plummet because of "overutilization." Or the added costs may come out of your own pocket, in a variety of ways. On the other hand, if you deny the patient's request because the situation doesn't warrant the particular test or specialist referral they insist on, you may receive a phone call from the patient representative, telling you that your decision has been overturned in the patient's favor. Why? The patient complained.

These are just a few of the many stresses and frustrations we hear about weekly as we travel around the nation, working with physicians and other health care professionals. It is not hard to see the discouragement and frustration on their faces. Many are leaving the profession, depressed and angry that they can't practice the kind of medicine they envisioned when they entered training years ago.

That is what has prompted this book. With all the talk about patient satisfaction, perhaps it's time to also take a look at *your own* satisfaction. How could you go home more satisfied with patient interactions, more relaxed, and with a greater sense of professional satisfaction at the end of the day?

The techniques and tips in this book will help you do just that. Although we can't increase the amount of time you have with patients, we can show you how to use that time to greater advantage—and in a way that helps your patients perceive their time with you as longer than it actually is. We can't change the attitudes or the personalities of your challenging patients, but we can show you some unique ways to handle them, some new approaches that will help reduce the tension and improve the relationship.

If you are prepared with a variety of proven techniques to manage the communication glitches in your day, you are likely to feel less stressed and more positive. You'll have more energy to bring your full array of talents and abilities into your practice. It was, after all, your interest in helping others that brought you into medicine—or at least it was a significant factor. We hope *Communicating with Today's Patient* supports that worthy purpose.

PRACTICAL, USEFUL ADVICE

The studies by top medical communications researchers cited throughout this book present valuable information that can significantly improve your interactions with patients. But when I report these research findings to clinicians in communication workshops, they often say, "OK, but how do you *do* that? You've just told us that 'Good listening skills are associated with patients having a higher assessment of quality care.' I think I *do* listen and *do* show an interest in my patients. Give us some concrete examples of what 'good listening' looks and sounds like." That's exactly the goal of this book.

We take the findings of research in medical communication to the next step, offering specific examples of how you can incorporate them into your daily interactions with patients. This book is a self-help manual of clinical communication skills, based on the excellent research in medical communications that is available today. We hope that this book will prove to be a handy resource that you can refer to regularly in the years to come.

A QUICK FIX?

These tips and techniques provide a sort of topical application in the form of useful phrases and practical suggestions you can quickly master to make your interactions with patients more effective and more efficient. Although it's true that attitude, commitment, and practice are what bring about the most profound changes in behavior, the value of our skills-based approach is summed up in an old saying: "You can't think your way into a new way of acting, but you can act your way into a new way of thinking." As a communication coach, I have seen this happen often over the years.

WHO CAN BENEFIT FROM THIS BOOK

If you have had any feedback from patients—ever—that you don't seem to listen or don't seem to be caring enough (or if you've had that feedback from your spouse, partner, or friend), this book can provide specific ways to be more expressive and to demonstrate clearly that you are listening and that you do care.

Others who can benefit from this book are those clinicians who, although highly adept at listening and quite comfortable with expressing their feelings, nevertheless often feel uncomfortable or even upset by challenging, demanding patients, and frequently run behind schedule as a result. If you are stressed by patients who seem angry and difficult, who don't follow your recommendations, or who lodge complaints about you, we have suggestions for how you can communicate with them more successfully. These techniques will leave you both feeling far less stressed, more respectful of each other, and more satisfied on the whole.

In addition, this book can be helpful to anyone who spends the majority of the day interacting with patients: physicians, physician assistants, dentists, nurses and nurse practitioners, medical assistants, front-office and back-office staffs, and hospital workers. Daily communication hassles, even when they are relatively minor, have cumulative effects, causing major stress. The communication approaches in this book are helpful in reducing those routine irritations in your busy day.

WHAT YOU'LL GET FROM THIS BOOK

Each chapter is full of what the physicians and other clinicians in our workshops have called "communication pearls." *Communicating with*

Today's Patient is not intended to be an all-inclusive, weighty tome of research and theory. We also realize that some parts are more useful for you than others, depending on your particular practice specialty and setting. For example, we do not cover skills dealing with very specialized types of patients, such as those dependent on drugs or alcohol or those who have serious mental health problems. Rather, the skills in this book apply to the majority of patients whose personalities and problems lie basically within the standard bell curve of patients in a primary care practice. Those 5–15 percent at either end are beyond the scope of this book and require specialized input from experts in those fields.

HOW THIS BOOK IS ORGANIZED

In Chapter One, we cover the many advantages that accrue from effective communications—a host of clinical benefits that are clearly associated with positive patient interactions.

Chapter Two looks at essential communication skills for quickly establishing a good relationship with each new patient—and for reinforcing your relationships with existing patients. Strong patient relationships are the foundation stones of any successful practice.

Understanding the personalities of your patients is the topic of Chapter Three; emphasis is on the personality styles you may find most frustrating. Step-by-step approaches—such as strategies to defuse angry patients and useful phases you can employ—are included to help you manage and perhaps even begin to feel more positive about these challenging interactions. The worst time to try to figure out rationally what to do is when you're in the middle of a fray, facing a challenging patient. By using the strategies in this book, you are better prepared for those difficult situations that inevitably come along.

Chapter Four focuses on body language, which often speaks so loudly it can drown out your words. Some important do's and don'ts are included so that you can avoid sending any mixed messages or unintended put-downs of your patients or colleagues.

Chapter Five covers listening skills, which include listening for covert as well as overt messages from patients. Since good listening depends on skillful questioning, we also look at question formats that can reveal the patient's real story faster and more accurately to help in making your final diagnosis.

Clear explanations are essential to compliance (or the term we prefer, adherence). Chapter Six offers an array of useful techniques for giving patients a clear understanding of their treatment plans. This is one of the longest chapters, since your explanations not only have an impact on your quality of care and patient outcomes but can also save you considerable time and expense over the years.

Chapter Seven focuses specifically on explanations about medications, since this has a profound effect on adherence and patient outcomes.

In surveys conducted with clinicians attending Desmond Medical Communications workshops, a problem that is often mentioned is dealing with patients' family members. In Chapter Eight we cover a variety of approaches you can use with family members to turn them from possible adversaries into probable allies in the important task of managing your patient's care.

Chapter Nine covers issues related to communicating with patients from diverse ethnic backgrounds.

Finally, your professional image is the topic of Chapter Ten. It often influences whether patients choose you and whether they stay with you. This chapter is well worth your time since it has important information for everyone on your staff as well. Good impressions can make or break your ties with patients.

The tips and techniques in all the chapters reflect practical, day-to-day communication skills that anyone working in health care needs to have at the ready, to deal effectively and efficiently with the large number of patients seen each week. The communication skills we share in this book chiefly address the art of medicine, which helps you practice the science of medicine, so that the business of medicine can support your art and science.

WHERE THESE COMMUNICATION PEARLS COME FROM

The majority of the skills covered in this book have been taught for fifteen years in Desmond Medical Communications' patient communication workshops presented throughout the United States. Other skills have been taught for twenty years in our presentation skills workshops. Some are techniques learned from experience in the world of media; some come from academia through our formal training. But many of the best pearls come from experienced physicians and other health care professionals whom we have been privileged to work with over the years. The pearls these talented communicators have shared with us add a special luster to this collection.

We also drew, in part, on the materials used in the medical schools and residency training programs at Harvard University School of Medicine, the University of Michigan Medical School, and several other institutions. Classes in communication are now becoming a regular part of the medical curriculum; many of tomorrow's clinicians will graduate well schooled in patient communications.

OUR GOAL: SOLUTIONS

This book gives you time-proven, road-tested communication techniques. Adjust them to fit your style. Skip over any you're already using. Apply them according to your own best medical instincts. Practice the ones you need for a crisis, so that you have them at the ready. And, of course, PRN—take as needed.

Chicago, Illinois   Joanne Desmond
Albany, Georgia   Lanny R. Copeland, M.D.
July 2000

ACKNOWLEDGMENTS

Many people contributed to this book, including my coauthor, Lanny Copeland, who, despite his dizzying schedule as president of the American Academy of Family Physicians, was able to bring to these pages his medical expertise and many years of experience as a successful, practicing physician, as an academician, and as a leader in today's health care. His insights have been invaluable. My thanks also to colleagues Margaret DeFleur; Kirk Strawn, M.D.; Alan Woolf, M.D.; Helene Klein Finestein; Susan Keane Baker; and Ron Pickett, as well as to Margaret, Scott, Rick, and Michael Easley, all of whom helped make this book possible.

But surely the greatest debt is owed to my friend and colleague Donald Gancer, who brought his extensive literary background to the task of editing and advising me, steadfastly at my side throughout the entire process of writing this book. He receives my heartfelt gratitude for his constant encouragement and diligent help in bringing this book to print.

Joanne Desmond
President
Desmond Medical Communications

CHAPTER 1

Ten Reasons You Need to Read This Book

You will probably conduct between 100,000 and 160,000 patient interviews during the course of your clinical career, according to a report by Linda Nichols and David Mirvis, M.D. (1998, p. 94). With this kind of volume, taking steps to be certain that you derive the fullest benefits from those interactions, day after day, is a reasonable precaution. The communication techniques in this book ensure the best use of those thousands of hours that still lie ahead for you.

Learning new information has probably always come easily to you. But intellect and technical brilliance are quite distinct from a talent for successful professional and social interactions. Skill at communicating, which often needs to be studied and practiced for many years, may have less to do with your intellectual abilities than with your emotional abilities.

TEN BENEFITS OF IMPROVED COMMUNICATION SKILLS

One has never "finally arrived" at being a good communicator. It is an ongoing process, with plenty of bumping into walls and course-correcting. Communication skills need constant sharpening, particularly in an environment where complexity and stress levels are high. But regularly tuning up your communication style with patients can reap a host of benefits. Here are ten reasons to read this book—ten advantages awaiting you within these pages.

1. More Accurate Diagnoses

Your skills in questioning and listening are critical to making an accurate diagnosis, since as many as 76 percent of final diagnoses are based on getting the patient's history (Peterson and others, 1992).

Using the listening techniques recommended in Chapter Five can help you unlock your patient's secrets. Skillful questioning, coupled with appropriate responses, can also give you deeper understanding of the complexity of the patient's illness (Rosenberg, Lussier, and Beaudoin, 1997). "When your patient senses, 'Here's someone I can really talk to, someone who will listen and understand me,' that patient is more likely to open up, to be comfortable telling you embarrassing or emotional experiences of illness. That relationship is most important in the personal care of the patient today," says John D. Stoeckle, M.D., Harvard Medical School. Such open communication is often an essential ingredient in making an accurate diagnosis.

Along the same lines, if patients keep their hidden concerns hidden, it often leads to the last-minute blurting out of those dreaded words, "Oh, while I'm here, I just thought I'd mention . . ." and other variations of the "oh-by-the-way" theme. The listening skills covered in Chapter Five include several techniques for getting those patients with hidden agendas to open up earlier, which can significantly improve the accuracy of your diagnosis.

2. Time Savings

That last-minute "Oh, by the way" can cost a significant amount of lost time in your busy day. If the last-minute concern suddenly introduces new and serious health issues, it often brings an exasperated sigh from the clinician and an internalized moan of "Why didn't you tell me that earlier?!" In Chapter Five there are a number of question formats you can use to be sure you get the real presenting complaint, the often hidden one that actually brought the patient to see you in the first place. Using these techniques can save you from vigorously pursuing the wrong problem for the entire visit, or from having to schedule another visit for the patient.

Approximately forty clinicians who had attended Desmond Medical Communications workshops were asked if they saved time by using the skills learned. Sixty-eight percent reported affirmatively, and several even said they had saved an estimated two to four hours a week. The participants were primary care physicians, physician assistants, and nurse practitioners, all in managed care plans and all polled anonymously. Many of the same time-saving communication techniques that we cover in our workshops are found throughout this book.

If a patient lodges a complaint, it can cost at least an hour of administrative time—usually on the part of an office manager or, if the doctor works for a larger health care organization, a patient representative. Complex complaints, which come in from other avenues (including those from executive offices, local or state agencies such as the board of medical examiners, or a senator's office), can require far more time. Depending on the number of staff involved and the time it takes, settling a patient complaint can cost hundreds or even thousands of dollars. One colleague who works with a large managed care organization reports that some formal complaints can cost up to $20,000. An even greater cost to a medical group or health plan comes from giving patients unnecessary referrals or tests and procedures in order to appease them. However, the greatest potential financial loss occurs if the patient switches to another health care plan or medical practice.

"But," you might respond, "it takes time to use this patient-focused approach! I only have ten to fifteen minutes per patient as it is. Take time to listen to their emotional concerns? Get real!" The reality is that in most cases it does not require significant additional time (Roter and others, 1997). Researchers have also found that even when talk centers largely around psychosocial issues, the length is not appreciably longer than for other visits. In still other studies, some of the visits in which the patients' emotional concerns were dealt with were actually shorter (van Dulmen, Verhaak, and Bilo, 1997).

Through timing the role plays in Desmond Medical Communications workshops over the past fifteen years, it has become clear that using the skills we recommend can give the person sitting in the patient's seat the perception that the interaction with the clinician is longer than is actually the case. To you, time is real and rationed, counted in precious seconds and minutes. But to patients, time is a perception, counted in warm smiles and murmurs of understanding.

3. Greater Patient Retention

Whether patients stay with you over the years or switch to someone else correlates strongly with how well you communicate with them (Gordon, Baker, and Levinson, 1995). Physicians and other clinicians who were better communicators had fewer appointments canceled by patients and had more patients coming in to see them (DiMatteo, Hays, and Prince, 1986). A 1995 survey by *Medical Economics* showed that as many as 44 percent of patients said they left their physicians because of something the physician said or did; yet only 27 percent said they'd leave for cheaper insurance (Slomski, 1995). Clearly, a good bedside manner has high value in patients' estimation. For specific techniques that are especially effective for maintaining patient loyalty, see Chapter Three on patient personalities and Chapter Four on body language.

4. Greater Satisfaction—for You and Your Patients

As we said in the Preface, this book was prompted in large part by an interest in helping physicians and other clinicians gain a greater sense of professional satisfaction. Warm, humanistic interactions with your patients and with their families can be gratifying and uplifting for you as well as for your patients. The techniques suggested within these pages can make your days more interesting and more fulfilling.

In terms of patient satisfaction, studies indicate that the clinician's skill in communicating can significantly affect the number of complaints from patients, the degree of overall patient satisfaction, and retention of existing patients (Gordon, Baker, and Levinson, 1995). If you show patients that you are interested in listening to the emotional aspects of their illness and can empathize with them, their satisfaction increases significantly (Bertakis, Roter, and Putnam, 1991). You create a powerful connection or bonding with the patient that is not likely to be jeopardized or strained by the patient through such discordant action as lodging a complaint to the office manager or other administrator. Throughout this book, you will find effective techniques for showing patients that you are interested in hearing their psychosocial concerns as well as their physical complaints. Be sure to check Chapters Four and Five in particular.

5. Increased Patient Compliance

Compliance, or the term we prefer—adherence—generally increases if patients are given clear and understandable information about their condition and progress in a sincere and responsive way, and if the physician elicits and respects patients' concerns (Becker, 1985). This is not the case, however, if the information is given in an abstract, academic manner. Chapter Six has tips for giving clear, jargon-free explanations to your patients, which several studies indicate is strongly associated with greater patient adherence to the prescribed treatment plan and the medications you recommend (Becker, 1985). Effective communication skills have also been shown to promote patients' increased satisfaction with their care, greater adherence to treatment regimens, and improved response to the treatment itself (Bertakis, Roter, and Putnam, 1991; DiMatteo, 1994; Grüninger, 1995).

In addition, if patients sense through the way you communicate that you care about them as individuals, they are more likely to make a leap of faith and assume that everything you do is probably in their best interest. This kind of generalized buy-in from patients tends to extend to other recommendations you make to them thereafter, such as the medications you prescribe, the treatment plans and procedures, and even the surgery you advise. For specific ways to achieve such acceptance from your patients, see Chapters Two and Three in particular.

6. Better Patient Outcomes

Research has established that there is definitely a relationship between how physicians and patients behave during an office visit and the patients' subsequent health status. In her overview of several important studies on the topic, Moira Stewart points out that effective communication can exert a positive influence not only on the emotional health of the patient but also on symptom resolution, functional and physiologic status, and pain control (Stewart, 1995). Patients whose physicians were less controlling and responded to the patients' questions with more information during the baseline visit showed improved health status at follow-up, measured both by functional status and by the patients' self-reports (Kaplan, Greenfield, and Ware, 1989).

At forty-two intensive care units throughout the nation, researchers found that caregiver interaction was significantly associated with lower risk-adjusted length of stay and greater efficiency in terms of moving patients in and out of an ICU. In addition, the patients thought their technical quality of care was better, and they even believed the needs of family members were better met (Shortell and others, 1994). A whole bundle of benefits can be derived from effective communication!

7. Higher Marks for Quality of Care

As is the case with adherence, if patients believe that you sincerely like them and want the best for them, they tend to assume that all your efforts on their behalf are of the highest quality. Patients are far more likely to assess your quality of care as "high" if they think you communicate well with them. Friendly, engaging caregivers tend to be perceived by their patients as having superior clinical skills. However, this does not eclipse clinical competence. Just being nice or caring without showing thoroughness and competence in the medical tasks is not enough to inspire confidence in patients or in the quality of care they receive (Hall, Roter, and Katz, 1988).

Quality is one of the important criteria for gaining accreditation and for meeting national standards for quality of care. Patients' input regarding their perceived quality of care is an increasingly important factor in both. In addition, such patient assessments of quality constitute a powerful marketing tool for promoting your individual practice or organization, often proving to be your competitive edge.

We have been called in by a number of clients prior to NCQA reviews. (The National Committee for Quality Assurance is a Washington-based organization that accredits managed care organizations.) The resulting workshops, with individual coaching in patient communication techniques, always significantly improve the organization's patient satisfaction scores. Follow-up patient satisfaction surveys showed that in many cases the improvement was as high as 40–50 percent. A concerted effort to improve interactions with patients, coupled with specific communication techniques, can have a rapid and profound impact on patient satisfaction assessments.

8. Reduced Risk of Malpractice

A number of studies indicate that poor communication may be a more important factor than poor outcome in predicting litigation. A study of malpractice depositions indicated that communication problems between the physician and patients were identified in 70 percent of cases (Beckman, Markakis, Suchman, and Frankel, 1994). A team of researchers led by Wendy Levinson, M.D., found that primary care physicians with no malpractice claims used specific communication approaches more frequently than did physicians who had a history of claims. These communication techniques included checking for understanding, educating patients about what to expect during their visit, and encouraging patients to talk (Levinson and others, 1997).

Two other researchers who also delved into causes of malpractice, Gregory Lester and Susan Smith, sum up their findings: "The results of our study support the idea that physicians may be able to affect their risk of lawsuits by changing the way they behave with patients. The use of good communication behaviors, for example, may not be technically more 'competent' medicine but it may prevent lawsuits, even when something has clearly gone wrong and even when it is clearly the physician's fault" (1993, p. 272). Improper performance of the diagnostic interview, evaluation, or consultation is the number one allegation against physicians in nearly all specialties, according to national data collected by the Physician Insurers Association of America (Sanders and McBride, 1998).

Maurice Garvey, a highly respected malpractice defense attorney in Chicago, told us, "Many lawsuits begin long before the alleged act of malpractice occurs." He added, "If you relate well to your patients, take the time to talk with them and with their families in a caring way, that's a major step in reducing your malpractice risk." Several years ago, I presented a program on how to avoid malpractice litigation with Alice Gosfield, past president of the National Health Lawyers Association (now the American Health Lawyers Association). She told me, "The data shows and I have also seen from my own experience that patients don't sue physicians they sincerely like and trust."

So, how do you get patients to like and trust you? Chapters Two and Four in particular list a number of practical suggestions for forging a strong and enduring relationship. As we stated earlier, an added advantage is that most of the techniques won't take any extra time from your busy day—and many may actually save you time in the long run. Also, be sure to check Chapter Three on dealing with various personalities, Chapter Five on listening, and Chapters Six and Seven on giving explanations patients will understand, remember, and follow. All of them cover additional risk-reducing, patient-pleasing techniques that you can begin using at once.

9. A Thriving Medical Practice

We have observed that to have a successful practice any clinician must have three core competencies: the science, the art, and the business of medicine. In years of working with medical groups throughout the nation, we have seen individual practices as well as entire organizations that had one or two of the competencies but lacked a third. If all three competencies are not fully functioning as part of the culture, the practice or organization invariably fails to thrive—or is absorbed by another, stronger organization that has all three firmly in place.

10. Tune Up Personal and Professional Communications

You're probably thinking, at some level, "I really don't need this. I communicate just fine with my patients." Of course. That's how many clinicians see it, especially those who are physicians. A number of studies, notably by Richard Street, Jr., and John Wiemann (1988), conclude that physicians tend to think they communicate far better than their patients think they do. In fact, the studies indicated that physicians' self-assessments are dramatically different from their patients' perceptions. Physicians also tend to believe they don't use jargon, yet studies show they do and don't realize it (Korsch, Gozzi, and Francis, 1968). So, factoring in that you may be predisposed to overestimate your own communication effectiveness, there are probably a lot of suggestions in this book that you will find useful and that your patients will no doubt appreciate as well.

PUTTING IT ALL INTO PRACTICE—YOUR PRACTICE

The ten reasons for reading this book may provide motivation, but it's still up to you to incorporate the communication tips we recommend into your repertoire of clinical skills for daily use. Here are a few important points to keep in mind as you do that.

Communication Skills Can Be Learned

From my own experience as a medical communications coach, as well as from a considerable body of research, it's clear that communication skills can be learned. If you were given some golf balls and a bag of clubs and told to just go and play, with no coaching on the techniques involved in a good swing, for example, it's not likely that you would become a skilled golfer.

Similarly, appropriate communication and interviewing techniques are best learned with a structured approach, including specific techniques and coaching, and not just informally or by chance through the experience of interacting with a large number of patients. Frederick Wolf, assistant professor of postgraduate medicine and health professions education at the University of Michigan, and his research associates corroborate the need for structured learning of communication skills (Wolf, Wooliscroft, Calhoun, and Boxar, 1987).

Levinson and Roter also measured the effects of communication training for physicians and found it beneficial in terms of improving participants' behaviors (1993). True, some are just "born communicators." But we have seen many clinicians who were not born with a special talent for communication nevertheless successfully master the skills—some quite easily, others with disciplined practice. They learned and improved, and so can we all.

Communication Can't Be Delegated

"I've got a really friendly nurse," a busy surgeon recently stated in a workshop. "She takes care of all that stuff like worried patients and the weepers— so I can get on with things. She's really great at that. I just let her handle 'em." The surgeon revealed later that he was attending the workshop because he'd just been named as a defendant in his first malpractice suit and wanted to "get a few tips" on how to communicate better.

The reality is, the buck stops with you. The responsibility for communicating can't be passed on to a friendly nurse or a schmoozy partner. Your patients want a caring, committed relationship with you. It's their guarantee that you will always give them your best effort—even if they're anesthetized on an operating table.

Communication Is an Essential Clinical Skill

"It may seem natural to achieve therapeutic success by placing great emphasis on physical exams, x-rays, sonograms, medications and surgeries," says researcher Robin DiMatteo (1994, p. 149) of the University of California at Riverside. But studies indicate that when this is done to the exclusion of a meaningful exchange of information and ideas, or without understanding and respect for the autonomy of the patient, several critical elements of patient care and treatment quality are adversely affected (DiMatteo, 1994).

Even a Few New Techniques Can Make a Big Difference

If you take away half or even a fourth of these communication techniques, you will notice significant improvements in your interactions with patients in the coming months and years. We are convinced that reading and incorporating at least some of the tips and insights presented here will prove well worth your effort.

If you think that communication techniques associated with getting a better diagnosis, improving patient outcomes, increasing the probability of patient adherence, growing your practice, managing your tight schedule, and reducing your malpractice risk are worth your time and attention, this book will prove invaluable.

We start out, in the next chapter, by catching a new patient just coming through the front door of your office or clinic. We offer a checklist of communication techniques you can use—right from that first visit—to keep this patient, and others, coming back through your doors for many years to come.

CHAPTER 2

Tips to Keep New Patients and Build Your Practice

I n this chapter, we highlight how you can quickly forge a bond with those new patients who show up in your exam room. Retaining each new patient who walks in the door takes on added importance if your goal is to grow your practice and avoid the turnover of patients affecting so many clinicians today. Although the primary effort is always to better serve the patient, the skills covered here are also effective in building your practice, stabilizing your patient base, and reducing the churn, one patient at a time.

Patient turnover is a significant problem because when a patient leaves your practice, it not only disrupts continuity of care for the patient but also represents lost income to you. An article in *Group Practice Journal* points out that the finding from customer service research that it costs five times more to acquire a new client than to keep an existing client has significant ramifications for the health care setting as well (Luecke, Rosselli, and Moss, 1991). The cost of acquiring a new patient is approximately seven times greater than that of keeping a patient you already have, judging by customer service research (Luallin and Sullivan, 1998). Yet today it's a daunting task to retain existing patients and keep them happy, especially in an era when patients are more outspoken about their health care than they used to be, more informed (as well as misinformed), increasingly litigious, and less likely to be loyal. To compound the problem, the time you have for establishing a relationship with new patients—or for nourishing relationships with existing patients—is squeezed.

The Norman Rockwell scenes of the family doctor who has time to engage in long conversations with a family he's taken care of for three generations, or to sew up a young patient's sick teddy bear, are still within the experience of anyone over fifty. These views of the comfortable family doctor remain a strong part of the nation's medical tradition and are still the ideal against which many people measure health care delivery. This will remain the case for decades to come.

Despite the hurdles of today's competitive health care market, your efforts to keep more patients can pay off mightily.

FIRST IMPRESSIONS COUNT

"How'd ya like Dr. Allen?" Beth calls out through the car window as she drops her youngsters at neighbor Carole's house.

Carole shrugs. "I don't know. Couldn't seem to connect. He's kinda distant." Herding the kids inside, she adds, "Definitely not the one for us."

Beth quickly leans out the window. "Really?! It *can* take a while to get to know him. But he's very knowledgeable. Oh well, Dee just loves Dr. Quinlan over on Fourth Avenue."

"Quinlan, huh?"

"Yeah. Give him a call. Be good, kids!"

She waves and drives off.

The Direct Cost of a Lost Patient

Carole's cryptic assessment of Dr. Allen will cost him approximately $10,819 in direct revenue loss, according to Luecke, Rosselli, and Moss (1991). But aside from the dollar cost of losing a new patient, there is also the missed opportunity of having Carole and her family as patients whom Dr. Allen might have enjoyed working with for many years.

The Indirect Cost of a Lost Patient

Dr. Allen's professional reputation is also likely to suffer, since, in addition to Beth, Carole will probably tell nine or ten others about her disappointment with him. In fact, Luecke, Rosselli, and Moss (1991) say that ultimately as many as sixty-seven others may indirectly hear negative word-of-mouth information about Dr. Allen, which might influence them not to use that physician or practice. Factoring all this in, the same researchers put the figure for potential lost revenue from one dissatisfied patient at approximately $238,018. In health care, word of mouth can be the most rewarding, or the most damaging, marketing tool of all.

What You Don't Know Can Hurt You

Ironically, Carole won't tell Dr. Allen about her dissatisfaction; approximately three out of ten patients don't do so (Goodman, 1999). The fact that Carole's first impression was negative would have been useful information for Dr. Allen. But how can he fix what he doesn't know is broken?

Carole's reaction may be just the tip of the iceberg. If Dr. Allen comes to understand that his demeanor with patients needs attention, he might face that; seek help through coaching, classes, or books; and make improvements that can help him keep other patients. Complaints are not just downers to make you feel incompetent; they are valuable signals to be heeded—directional markers along your professional pathway, and guides to improvement.

First Impressions Happen Fast!

Patients begin making their initial assessments of you within the first few seconds of seeing you. When you walk into the room, patients begin receiving your nonverbal messages at a subliminal level, before you even open your mouth to say, "How can I help you today?" As you talk with them, your words and your style of expression also come under patients' intuitive scrutiny, although they may not be entirely aware of how carefully they are taking your measure.

Is it really fair for Carole or any patient to make a final judgment about the professional abilities of a clinician based on a few impressions from one short meeting? Of course not. But do they? Of course. So, when you walk into the exam room to see a new patient, keep in mind that if the first impression you make on that patient is not a good one, it will probably be the last one.

IMPORTANT FACTORS AFFECTING PATIENTS' CHOICES

What does a patient look for when determining who will deliver high-quality care? From current research, we now know quite a lot about how that process works.

The Decision Maker's Viewpoint

The key person who decides which primary care clinician the family goes to is likely to be a wife or mother. Women make at least 75 percent of the consumer health care decisions in the United States, according to sources cited in *Megatrends for Women* (Aburdene and Naisbitt, 1992).

When I was chosen to be the host of the prime-time medical talk program "Doctors' House Call," it was largely because I was a middle-aged female with a family, and therefore typical of the average decision maker on health care services.

Since patients have many more choices about their health care today, they do what they always do when the decision is important: they shop around and compare. Whether it's a new house, new car, new dentist, or new physician, they check out the options. You would too.

Many patients use Carole's method to find a suitable clinician: word-of-mouth recommendation, often talking to only one or two friends or family members rather than asking other health care professionals for recommendations. The positive reports of others, including neighbors and family members, who've had experience with a particular physician seem to count heavily—as much as 50 percent—in the final decision. Word-of-mouth recommendations may be twice as influential as other advertising approaches (Goodman, 1999).

Your Competitive Edge

Since patients generally assume that most physicians will know how to diagnose what is wrong and prescribe what is needed, the differentiating factor in building market share is service, according to health care consultants Luallin and Sullivan (1998). In a patient survey on loyalty conducted by *Medical Economics*, the percentage of patients who reported that they left a practice over something a doctor or the doctor's staff did or said to them was as high as 44 percent. The main reason cited by respondents was their perception that the doctor was arrogant and talked down to patients in a patronizing way. Impersonal treatment and rudeness were other common reasons given for abandoning a doctor, according to this study (Slomski, 1995). It is interesting to note that research on the factors leading to malpractice indicates that these same patient perceptions are also key reasons that patients bring lawsuits.

Patients' Priorities

The number one benefit most patients are looking for costs you nothing out of pocket—not even more of your time, in many cases. The overwhelming factor in choosing a particular physician or clinician—for 84 percent of patients, according to those surveyed—was how well a clinician communicates and whether or not the clinician shows a caring attitude—both of which we think fit under the umbrella of good patient communication (Engstrom and Madlon-Kay, 1998).

A 1996 survey of 12,000 health care consumers by a large Midwestern HMO asked which factors were most important in patients' decisions to stay or leave (Luallin and Sullivan, 1998). Those that addressed physician-patient communication included, in order of importance, the following:

- Giving clear explanations and instructions
- Answering patients' questions sufficiently and appropriately
- Spending time with patients
- Showing concern for patients
- Giving test results to patients in a timely manner
- Being courteous on the telephone
- Warm, friendly nurses and staff
- Explaining the reason for delays

Here are other criteria that patients find important in deciding which physician or plan to go with, according to a 1996 national survey cosponsored by the Agency for Health Policy and Research and the Kaiser Family Foundation and reported by Engstrom and Madlon-Kay (1998):

- Board certification was important to 71 percent of the patients.

- Number of years in practice was important to 35 percent.

- Having attended a well-known medical school or training program was valued by 30 percent.

Other factors such as age, gender, marital status, or languages spoken seemed far less important to the patients surveyed.

The Most Popular Perks

Convenient parking, discounts at a local movie house or health club, and money-back guarantees if they're not seen on time are appreciated by patients. The most popular perks, however, according to a patient attitude survey published in *Medical Economics* (Weber, 1995), are free beverages in the waiting room, a patient newsletter, and brochures or videos on health care topics to peruse while they are waiting to be seen. Whatever perks you offer, patients no doubt appreciate your thoughtfulness and the expense you've gone to in order to please them.

Changing Priorities of Today's Patient

It's interesting to note that board certification carries so much weight in patient choices today, since only about twenty years ago many patients didn't know what *board certified* meant or thought it wasn't an important indicator of a physician's skill level. As medical topics increasingly appear in the popular media and thus educate patients through articles and news broadcasts, patients are becoming more discriminating consumers about choosing their physician and their health care plan.

Form and Substance Are Both Important

Patients are no longer satisfied with just a soothing bedside manner. They want substance in terms of clinical skills. Highly respected researchers in medical communications believe that a clinician's ability in performing medical tasks, such as giving clear explanations, can indicate to his or her patients that the clinician cares about the patient and values the person as an individual

(Hall, Roter, and Katz, 1988). We agree, and this is why we devote much of this book to specific communication techniques that can be incorporated directly into clinical skills—for example, techniques for listening to get an accurate diagnosis, explaining so that the patient adheres to the regimen, and so forth.

The Importance of Patients' Perceptions

At the same time, many patients also rely heavily on their own intuitive, gut-level, affective responses to you. Their assessment of the quality of your care is often heavily weighted by how well you *seem* to communicate with them, their *perception* of how much you care about them, and whether they *feel* you will always provide a safe haven for their emotional as well as physical concerns (Desmond, 1990).

These patient perceptions of you can make or break your new relationship. How skillfully you communicate can outweigh all your academic credentials, framed and proudly hanging on the wall. An old saying makes the point: "They don't care how much you know—until they know how much you care."

What Can You Do?

If good first impressions are so important in keeping new patients, then it's valuable to know specifically what you can do to increase the probability that a first meeting goes well—what you can do to increase the likelihood of keeping that new patient, someone like Carole. Ideally, not only the patient but also the patient's family and friends will become loyal patients in the long run. Are there some specific techniques you can use so that new patients have a positive feeling about you right off the bat?

Sure, there are. Skillfully implemented, these techniques can be potent factors in ensuring that a new patient keeps coming back for many years.

GOOD OPENERS FOR THE NEW-PATIENT VISIT

Here are communication techniques that can significantly influence a patient's positive impression of you right from the first moments of that first appointment.

Pleasantly Surprise Patients by Not Barging In!

If you are like most clinicians, you knock on the door before entering the examination room in case the patient may be dressing. But we have found that, after knocking, very few clinicians actually wait for the patient's response. Most just enter when *they* are ready. This means the knock is really an announcement of intent to enter. If it is to be a polite query about the patient's readiness to be seen, the clinician should wait for the patient to signal that readiness by responding, "Come in." You would certainly observe knock-and-wait courtesy with anyone who was a guest in your home, so why not extend this same politeness to patients in your exam rooms? Waiting for the patient's OK to enter shows your respect, and it takes only an extra second or two.

In the hospital setting, it's difficult to observe this knock-and-wait courtesy, since patients are often sleeping, sedated, or curtained off. If the patient is in a room with a door that is open, it's courteous to at least knock on the doorframe and then come in and greet the patient. We're not suggesting this for nurses or medical assistants who have to pop in and out of a patient's hospital room frequently—for example, during post-op.

Slow Down! Don't Rush

Just before you enter the exam room or the hospital room, take a moment to slow down. It might prevent a costly error. Being rushed was one of the most frequently cited causes of physician error in a study conducted by Ely and others (1995). Slow your inner clock before greeting your patients, and, if you have been in a fast-paced mode all day, be sure to slow your speech when talking with them. If you don't, patients may quickly sense that you are in a hurry and resent the fact that you seem to be rushing them through the visit.

Some clinicians find it helpful to briefly roll their necks or quietly pause for a few seconds before entering an exam room. Others have found the relaxation techniques recommended by Dr. Herbert Benson (1975) helpful. They involve a few moments of deep abdominal breathing, concentrating on the sound of your own breathing, and just slowing your overall internal pace.

Have a Get-Acquainted Time

Take some time on that all-important first visit with a new patient. Close the chart and deliberately set it aside; allow no interruptions from the front office, from colleagues, or from the phone; and take a minute to just get to know the patient. Invite your new patient to tell you about his or her family, career, or other general information that is not directly related to the medical task. Lanny Copeland has successfully used this approach with new patients for many years and finds it invaluable for establishing a warm and caring relationship right at the start. It allows the patient to feel comfortable talking with you about many issues.

During this session, be sure that you also observe common courtesies, such as offering a place to hang a coat or hat or leave packages.

Give the Patient an Overview of the Visit

Early in the session, it helps to let your patient know the informal agenda for the visit, explaining what the general sequence will be. This need not take long. For example, you might say, "First I'd like to just talk with you, Mrs. Jones, and have the opportunity to know you better." Or "Right now, I'd like to hear about your health concerns. Then I'll examine you, and after that we can talk about where we go from there—what would be best for you." Or "After we discuss your health concerns, Mrs. Murray, I want to do a thorough examination, and then we'll have some time for any questions you may still have." This also gives the patient some orientation to the structure of the appointment.

Use Open-Ended Questions to Encourage Conversation

"What brought you in today?"

"A taxi."

There are always a few wags who give you that kind of answer, or variations on it ("My husband"). But the question is still a pretty good opener for a patient visit precisely because it's open-ended. The classic opener we like is, "How can I help you today?" Open-ended questions can't be answered with just a yes or a no. They invite and prompt a fuller answer. An open-ended question signals to patients that you are interested in hearing their "story" about their health concern.

This is a much better way to start off than beginning with a closed-ended question ("I understand you're having headaches. Did this just start?"). A closed-ended question subtly instructs the patient to be essentially passive, to follow your lead, and to respond only when you ask a question. It neither encourages a partnership nor invites the patient to open up to you. It can significantly affect how the patient views you: *abrupt, superior,* and *rushed* are impressions that are likely to come to a patient's mind. For more on the value of open-ended questions and the problems associated with closed-ended questions, see Chapter Five.

TIPS ON USING PATIENTS' NAMES

People love to hear their own name. Research tells us that right after you use a patient's name, you have that person's full attention for the next thirty seconds. Using your patients' names indicates your respect for them as important and unique individuals. It also indicates that you are courteous and will probably continue to be so throughout their relationship with you.

Check the Patient's Name and Use It

Before you go in to see the patient, take a moment to look at the chart and be sure you have the patient's name clearly in mind. Verify with the patient that you have the right name and that you pronounced it correctly.

A physician covering for a colleague rushed quickly into a post-op patient's hospital room, looked at the patient in the bed, pointed assertively, and began, "Mary, we need to . . . " The patient's husband irritably interjected, "Her name is *Dee.* Who are *you?*" Mary was asleep in the next bed.

No one in that room appreciated the young doctor's error. The story was told repeatedly in their small, closely knit community. It also hurt the hospital indirectly, since it implied that "the doctors there don't even know

Communicating with Today's Patient

or care who you are. They are so rushed that you'd better be careful they don't take out your gallbladder by mistake, or whack off a leg."

Use the Patient's Name Appropriately

There are two critical times to use the patient's name: at the beginning and at the end of the visit. That's a *minimum*. If you can gracefully and respectfully weave in the patient's name at other points in the interview, so much the better. Don't overdo it, of course, to the extent that you sound patronizing or obsequious.

The Patient's Name Gets Top Billing

In role plays during our workshops, clinicians often busily swish through the door, saying, "Good morning. I'm Dr. Swenson." Using this kind of introduction (which comes naturally enough to all of us), a caregiver can be perceived as superior and egotistical, since nothing indicates that the doctor knows or cares who the patient is.

Another version we often see is, "Good morning. I'm Dr. Swenson. I see Dr. Patel sent you." This kind of opening carries the implication that the only really important people to know are the two doctors, since they're the only ones mentioned. The patient may be left feeling like just another number or "the kidney stone in room 403."

Use the patient's name before your own: "Good morning, Mrs. Rodriguez. I'm Dr. Young" instead of "Good morning. I'm Dr. Young. Mrs. Rodriguez?"

Let's rerun that previous scenario. Rather than "Good morning. I'm Dr. Swenson. I see Dr. Patel sent you," a better version is, "Good morning, Mrs. Flynn, I'm Dr. Swenson. I'm happy to meet you. I see Dr. Patel sent you." Try to use the patient's name before your own, and also before the name of a referring clinician.

Do Patients Prefer Their First or Last Name?

Address patients by their last name and title until they indicate that they would like you to use their first name. Patients are often more willing to have you address them by their first names once they establish a relationship with you. However, certain groups tend to prefer always being addressed by their last name and title. According to studies by Gillette, Filak, and Thorne (1992), patients who have that preference are women and those who are nonwhite. Other studies corroborate this finding and add the group of people without commercial insurance (Dunn and others, 1987).

The answer as to what's best is not a simple one. But since a sizable portion of the patient population may be offended by being addressed by first name, the medical etiquette we recommend is to use last names unless the patients request that you use their first name (or a nickname).

A long-established relationship between clinician and patient in a small town or neighborhood where people know each other can make a big difference, of course, as to the appropriateness of using first names. Patients in a hospital or nursing home may prefer the closeness and familiarity of first-name usage, more so than "worried well" patients in an ambulatory clinic in a large metropolitan area.

One approach many clinicians use is to ask patients how they prefer to be addressed; this can be done with a questionnaire filled out at the first appointment. Once the information has been gathered, be sure it is entered into the patient's chart, where it can be used easily in all future introductions. It is often irritating to a patient to fill out a questionnaire and then find that the information they carefully wrote down has not even been read or entered into the system.

Use Titles Appropriately

Use the patient's title with the last name—*Mr., Mrs.* or *Ms., Judge, Colonel,* and so forth. Avoid addressing a female patient of any age as "young lady," "Hon," "Sweetie," or "Dear." Certainly do not say, "Hi, gorgeous," even as a good-natured joke. Though it's true some patients will like this, many will not. Those who don't like it tend to complain to administration or to the patient representative about being inappropriately addressed.

Professional women in particular often become incensed at this overly familiar approach, which they find patronizing and condescending. Over

Communicating with Today's Patient

the years, we've seen written complaints lodged against a number of health care clients.

Don't assume a woman is a "Mrs.," even if she is middle-aged. It can be quite insulting to a single woman to be addressed as "Mrs." when she is a "Ms." It implies an assumption about social norms that are no longer appropriate, or true, in society today.

Justices are addressed as "Judge" rather than "Your Honor," Catholic nuns are addressed as "Sister," and priests are addressed as "Father" rather than "Reverend." Rabbis are addressed as "Rabbi." Other clergy may wish to be addressed as "Reverend," but if you are in doubt, it is respectful to ask.

Avoid "Hey, You" Pronouns

Avoid using the third person singular pronoun when referring to the patient. Be careful not to say to a staff member, "Did you get her vitals?" or "Get him an appointment for an ultrasound, will you?" or "She needs an appointment for two weeks from now." No matter how rushed you are, try to use the patient's last name and title, even if you are talking about them down at the end of the hall. Using only the pronoun smacks of "Hey, you" and makes the patient feel faceless and unnoticed—just part of a hoard of patients, no one special.

Using the patient's name doesn't take any more time: "Did you get Mrs. Gold's blood pressure?" rather than "Did you get her blood pressure?" It may seem a small thing, but the effort pays off in the patient's sense of receiving individualized attention from you and your staff.

Pronounce the Patient's Name Correctly

If the patient's name is one that you might easily mispronounce or trip over, it should be written phonetically in the chart. Have a special place to do that, preferably right under the patient's printed name or nearby, so you and anyone else who may see the patient can be sure to pronounce the name correctly. Even if your patient charts are all on computer, there should still be a place for phonetic spelling of names on the computer records.

Writing names phonetically is simple. For example, Nguyen can be written as "Win," Beauchamps as "Bee-chum" (if the anglicized version of this French name is used), and Aguilar as "Ah-gee-lar." It's also important to show which syllable gets the emphasis, since this can affect correct pronunciation as well. Simply by using an apostrophe or by underlining that syllable—for example, Ah-kee-lar—you can indicate the stressed syllable.

It can be disconcerting to patients to hear their name called out in the waiting room in a mangled version. It's even worse if their name is still mispronounced on the third or fourth appointment. Correct pronunciation is courteous and sets a positive impression of respect and personal interest on the part of everyone on your clinic or office staff.

Greet Whoever Came with the Patient

If there are other family members or friends present with the patient, take a moment to turn to each, get his or her name, and acknowledge each of them. Shake hands if that seems appropriate. Acknowledging others who come with the patient is especially important with large, close families where the support of loved ones may be very important to the patient (as well as to the friend or family member).

When dealing with children or infants, of course, use the first name of the child who is your patient and the last name of the parent who comes with the child, since you are interacting directly with both in most cases. If the child is of preschool age or older, we suggest that you address the child first, then the parent or responsible adult.

Update Names Regularly

You can't assume that the last names of one family all match, even with a mother and small children. Nor can you assume that the last names stay the same over time. Yet you may be uncomfortable asking about this. One way you can determine last names is by focusing on the spelling: "I want to be sure the information we have in your chart is up-to-date and correct. So let's check that your names are spelled correctly in our records." Look

Communicating with Today's Patient

up expectantly and let the patient fill in. Do the same with family members present.

This allows you to be sure you are addressing patients and family members correctly; at the same time it keeps your chart information up-to-date. While doing this, it's also a good idea to check for next of kin, with updated telephone number and address. This can save hours of searching and telephoning in an emergency.

Be Aware of Cultural Issues When Greeting Patients' Families

For patients who are still tied closely to their Hispanic or Asian culture, family support is often associated in their health care beliefs with the patient's ability to recover from an illness. Individually greeting the other members of a family is courteous, respectful, and comforting to the patient.

Be sensitive to pecking order. With many multicultural families, including Asian and Hispanic families, it is frequently seen as appropriate to address the eldest of the family members first, beginning with the oldest male and then the oldest female. From there on, the hierarchical order usually runs through the generations of males and then of females. However, the reality is you may have to greet the rest of them according to their placement in the room, especially if there are several people in a small room and you're running behind schedule.

Introduce Yourself and Your Colleagues

When you or anyone on your staff introduces himself or herself to a new patient, use your title or state your position so the patient understands your role in his or her health care. Many times patients are embarrassed to ask what your position is; yet they may feel hesitant or uncomfortable talking to someone whose professional expertise they are not sure of. It's better to put that information right in your introduction: "Good afternoon, Captain Andrews, I'm Gail Swenson. I'm a physician assistant here, and I work with Dr. Habib. How can I help you today?"

In the hospital setting, you can say, "Good Morning, Mrs. Abrams, I'm Carolyn O'Leary. I'm a phlebotomist here at St. Joseph's. That means I've had special training for taking blood samples. I'll be taking your blood samples, usually in the mornings about this time. The samples give us a lot of important information which we need in order to give you the best care."

When you enter the room to meet with the patient, anyone else who is with you, such as a medical assistant, nurse, or resident, should also be introduced to the patient with a sentence about why the person is present for the interview. Again, in general use the patient's name first in your greeting; then introduce yourself, if necessary, and then your colleagues.

ESSENTIAL BODY LANGUAGE FOR A POSITIVE FIRST IMPRESSION

It takes less than a minute to make a patient feel valued. Since more than half of a positive attitude toward a patient is conveyed through your body language, here are some of the most essential of those silent messages.

Smile as You Say Hello

Smile when you greet the patient and the patient's family. It's an opportunity not to be missed. You may not have another chance to smile openly at the patient, since your demeanor is likely to be more serious as you listen to what he or she tells you during the history. A smile is one of the oldest and most universal ways of showing pleasure, throughout the world's cultures. It indicates clearly to patients that you're glad to see them and that you like them.

There are times, of course, when it is inappropriate to beam openly at the patient or the patient's family, particularly when dealing with serious illness. Rely on your own observations and instincts to tell you when a particular patient would prefer a more serious demeanor. But even if you don't smile fully and openly, your facial expression can match your verbal greeting. It is important to look pleased to see your patients—pleased to have the opportunity to work with them on their health issues.

Offer a Handshake If Appropriate

A handshake is generally accepted as appropriate touching; it is often a good way to start and end the visit.

Communicating with Today's Patient

Some patients are not comfortable with a handshake, so you will need to sense whether or not the patient is receptive. For example, older female patients or female patients from countries where the behavioral codes for women are quite distinct from those for men might be put off by an outstretched hand, especially one proffered by a male clinician.

Some patients, such as Asians, Indians, and Native Americans, who are still close to their cultural traditions may not feel entirely comfortable with a handshake, since it is not an integral part of their culture. Patients from what sociologists refer to as high-touch cultures, such as Hispanic and Mediterranean ones, tend to prefer some appropriate touching during the visit.

If you do shake hands with a patient of either gender, avoid what we call the hierarchical handshake: putting your other free hand on top of the patient's hand, sandwiching the patient's hand in the middle of your hands. Some patients may interpret this as your taking a position of superiority. However, we find that this sandwiching can be comforting to the patient in some cases, especially if you have your hands on both sides of the patient's hand.

Be Careful About Touching

In her book *That's Not What I Meant,* sociolinguist Debra Tannen states, "The doctor who pats his patient . . . on the arm, saying, 'How are you today, Sally?' may genuinely intend to be warm and friendly. But because the patient . . . couldn't pat him on the arm and ask, 'How are you today, Richie,' there's a (possibly unintended) metamessage of superior status in the doctor's gesture" (Tannen, 1986, p. 104).

Aside from whatever may be necessary during the examination, touching the patient has been shown to be a negative factor for patient satisfaction, especially on the first visit. Patients tolerate touching better after they establish a relationship with you.

Be sure that any touching, other than a handshake, is appropriate, such as what is necessary during the examination. You may also prefer that any touching of patients occurs only if another member of your staff is in the room with you.

Get the Color of the Patient's Eyes

Many clinicians tell us they always—absolutely always—have good eye contact as they talk to patients. Yet, when they are being videotaped in our workshop role plays, it is surprising how many don't! Physicians, pharmacists, dentists, and other clinicians, rushed for time, often don't realize they've fallen into the habit of glancing hurriedly at patients, or of not looking them in the eye at all, focusing instead on the chart, medication, or other impersonal objects. This is why we suggest that you note the color of each patient's eyes—perhaps even writing it in the chart. That way, you can be sure you looked directly in the patient's eyes at least once during the visit. Don't stare them down, just give them a frequent, sincere, eye-to-eye connection—especially when you or they are saying something important.

Check the Bridge of the Patient's Nose

If you feel uncomfortable looking into your patient's eyes, try a technique that TV reporters use during interviews. They look at the bridge of the person's nose if it is uncomfortable to look the person in the eye. To patients who like to receive this kind of attention, it will seem as if you are looking into their eyes, attentive and professionally interested in them. Of course, you don't want to stare them down. You can still look at the paperwork occasionally or at other points in the room. But if you are not used to looking people in the eye for several seconds at a time, this technique of looking at the bridge of the nose may prove helpful in getting started with making more eye contact.

Avoid the Cold Shoulder

Keep your shoulders squared toward the patient during your interactions. It tells the patient that he or she is your primary interest, not the chart or the medical task. We look at the importance of shoulder position more closely in Chapter Four. It's even more important, in some ways, than having good eye contact.

Flex a Few Facial Muscles

In a recent workshop role play, a physician's face was absolutely stoic throughout her entire videotaped explanation of a major surgical procedure that her "patient" would undergo in a few days. She had been expressionless throughout the entire day of the workshop, so I was not surprised to find this low affect in the role play as well. I discussed earlier in the class the need for some facial affect while listening or talking to the patient, but clearly she wasn't getting the message.

Finally, I decided to deal with it straight out. "Janet," I told her, "*Gray's Anatomy* says there are about four hundred muscles in the human face. Do you think you could move just one?" She actually smiled, and we determined that there was hope. Her facial muscles had not totally atrophied from lack of use.

Your facial expressions are an important part of your nonverbal communication and are being constantly and carefully monitored by your patients. It's a way patients read you to see if you are responsive, if you are someone they can relate to comfortably. We have more to say on facial expression and other body language in Chapter Four.

Focus on the Patient, Not the Chart

Be sure you don't turn away from the patient as you read the chart. Face the patient, with the chart angled to one side of you rather than placed between the two of you. We regularly observe clinicians putting the chart down on a table along the wall and reading it with their backs to the patient. Turning your back on the patient is . . . well, turning your back on the patient. It's cool and distant; it says, "I'm really only interested in the medical task here. The job I have to do is the most important thing, and you are only a necessary adjunct to that task."

An aging but popular actress whom we'll call Margaret recounted to us her recent visit to a dermatologist to determine whether she needed an acid peel or laser resurfacing of her still-beautiful face. She was seated in the examination chair awaiting the doctor. Suddenly, the door burst open and the nurse whisked past the chair, intently perusing the chart, without greeting or looking at Margaret.

The nurse laid the chart open on a counter at the back wall and efficiently read from it to verify the patient's name, dates of other surgeries, and the reason for this visit. Margaret sat in the chair facing forward; the nurse was behind her, facing in the opposite direction, curtly asking questions and writing in the chart. No possibility for eye contact. No facial expression to see. No warm, human interaction. It might as well have been done over an intercom!

Would this doctor's nurse be there to hold Margaret's hand and help her through the fear and possibly the pain involved in any of the procedures? Would the doctor? The nurse represented the entire practice as far as Margaret was concerned, and she quickly made a grand exit, stage right.

Room Layout Can Affect Communication

An office can be efficiently designed to provide care and yet inadvertently prevent good patient communication.

It's not just the body language and communication style of the nurse that's at fault in the previous example. The layout of the room encourages this style of interaction. A counter or desk attached to the back wall to hold the chart—or the computer display of the patient's chart—is not conducive to positive interactions with patients because it means the clinician's back is turned to the patient.

The only way there can be eye contact, and a chance to interact nonverbally as well as verbally, is if the room is set up so that the clinician can fully or at least partially face the patient.

After we pointed this out to a client who was medical director of a large managed care organization in Arizona, he had the clinicians' desks pulled off the back wall and repositioned in a way that was conducive to good eye contact and shoulder orientation between clinicians and patients. He later reported back to us that the new room arrangement made a significant difference in communicating, and everyone liked it much better.

SMALL TALK HAS A BIG PAYOFF

When you're double-booked and running late, the first casualty is often nonmedical chatting with the patient. But this can be one of your most effective ways to connect quickly with your patients.

Save a Few Moments for Small Talk

Engaging in a few moments of small talk helps set the patient at ease and establishes a common interest between the two of you. As we discussed earlier in this chapter, a get-acquainted time can be very effective. But in every visit, a few moments of small talk at the beginning and end make a nice transition. Studies indicate that patients tend to feel more satisfied with the interaction if there is a short chat period built in at the beginning. You don't need much time for this; even thirty to sixty seconds is often sufficient.

A little introductory small talk with your patients can be pleasurable for you as well, and it also significantly increases patients' perception of you as a pleasant, friendly person. While engaging in these few moments of small talk, be careful that your body language indicates that you are interested in what the patient is telling you. You lose the value of the time allowed for small talk (and actually turn it into a negative experience) if, while the patient is telling you about the thrill of visiting Hawaii last month, you have your back to the patient and are busily washing your hands in the sink.

Worse yet is reading the chart and muttering an occasional "Umhmm" as the patient tries to share treasured highlights. Setting aside time for small talk is valuable only if you show through your body language that you are truly interested in what the patient is saying.

Keep Track of Small-Talk Topics

As a corollary to the previous tip, have a place in the chart to jot down personal interests the patient tells you about as part of the opening small talk ("Just moved from Calif. Likes job—Misses sun" or "Proud of son's college scholarship" or, somewhat more cryptically written, "Hoop fan—esp. Chi. Bulls").

If you do this, you and the staff who see that patient know small-talk topics that have a high probability of delighting the patient, who is then likely to have the feeling "They all know me here!" This is especially important for patients who may be seeing various clinicians when they come in for appointments. There is more perceived continuity of care and a sense of comfort, since you all seem to know the patient at an individual level. The patient is not just being run through the mill or herded through like cattle, which are phrases we have seen in complaints lodged by patients in health care organizations.

SHARED LAUGHTER AND HUMOR

The role of humor in health care has gotten much play in recent years—from author Norman Cousins and from many practicing clinicians as well.

Laughter Lightens the Load

If patients tell you something they find amusing, be sure you take that opportunity for some shared laughter. A bit of laughter can lighten the patient's concerns, refresh the spirit, and even produce a few endorphins.

In terms of the clinician using humor with the patient, we tend to avoid specific recommendations because people vary so widely in their ability to use humor that it's difficult to give general tips. Humor can be extremely effective if used adroitly, but it is problematic if used inappropriately.

There are, however, a few guidelines for clinicians regarding the use of humor with patients. In general, avoid telling jokes to the patient. All humor should be what in theater they call an aside rather than an overt attempt to go for a laugh. This is humor that emanates naturally out of the situation, delivered in a light vein. You and the patient can both see the humor of the situation as equals, which allows you to bond. You probably have a few humorous lines that your patients consistently enjoy. But if you are not sure how well a bit of humor will go over or how appropriate it will be, consider the motto, "If in doubt, leave it out."

CLOSINGS

The final moments of the visit can cement the patient's perception of being cared for as a unique individual. And whatever happens at this point is likely to be remembered when the patient returns home.

Good Closings Make Good Beginnings

A few personal comments at the end of the visit, to show your interest in the patient as an individual, can bring the session to a warm close. You want the patient to leave your office feeling good about having spent time with you.

During those closing moments, it can be very effective to remember the last personal comments the patient shares with you, and jot them down. Next time you see the patient you can begin with, "When you were here last, you mentioned as you were leaving that you were going back home to start painting your kitchen. I hope that worked out well." Or "As we ended our last visit, you mentioned that you were leaving for Florida. I hope you had a good trip." It's very flattering to patients to know you care enough about them as individuals to remember these personal events, big or small. As we said earlier, small talk has a big impact on patient satisfaction and only takes a few seconds.

Have a Closing Ritual

The end of every patient visit should have a closing ritual that includes the following elements:

1. A well-wishing statement such as "I hope you'll be feeling better" or "I hope this medication gives us the results we want"

2. Using the patient's name again

3. Shaking hands, if it seems appropriate for this patient

4. Telling the patient where to go next, as needed: "Jane at the front desk can make your appointment for the tests we discussed today"

5. Saying you were pleased to have the opportunity to see the patient today

6. Being sure that you or someone sees the patient to the door and if possible even holds it open, especially for patients who might have trouble getting out

Here are just two examples of ways you can wrap the first five components into a few sentences. "I'm glad we were able to check this today, Mrs.

Smith. It was good to see you, and I look forward to seeing you again in two weeks." A pediatrician in one of our workshops has a favorite farewell: "I hope Johnny feels better soon, Mrs. Carter. It's hard having a sick child at home. I'd like to see you in two weeks to make sure his ears have improved, and I hope that he'll soon be feeling much better" (Desmond, 1995, p. 17). This is much more effective than just saying, "Come back in two weeks and we'll check him out."

Regarding seeing someone to the door, if the patient still needs to dress and you are not able to see her out, be sure someone at the front desk has the responsibility of seeing patients off with a warm farewell: "Good-bye, Ms. Jasinski, it was nice to see you today, and we look forward to seeing you again." Closings that leave the patient feeling cared about and cared for are actually openings of a new or renewed long-term relationship with you.

Don't let patients just drift away unnoticed. Even though it may be just another workday for you, going to see the doctor is a drama to many people. For you, the medical visit may start and end in the exam room or office. But for the patient, especially senior patients, the medical visit begins at home, with decisions about what to wear, what to remember to bring, and where to park; it ends when the patient returns home and talks with friends and family about what you said and did and what your information portends for the future.

The medical visit is an important, often dramatic event in a patient's life. It should have a ritual opening, elements of which we already discussed, and there should also be some sort of ritual farewell to wrap up the patient's visit, a finale that radiates warm, supportive, human interaction—a warmth the patient can still feel while walking to the parking lot or bus stop.

The various communication tools and tips in this chapter are helpful in getting off to a good start with a new patient, thereby increasing the probability of many future visits. If the patient does return, these skills are also highly effective in maintaining your relationships with existing patients.

In the next chapter, we look at the four main personality types of patients who show up in your exam room (both new and existing patients), and we cover some specific ways you can communicate smoothly with them, particularly when their personalities are quite different from yours.

CHAPTER 3

Patient Personalities and How They Affect Your Practice

Has this ever happened to you? You attend a meeting with a colleague and when it's over, you both walk down the hall discussing what happened. You listen to his opinion and think, "How could anyone possibly see it that way? I was right there, and it was completely different."

We all have distinct ways of viewing the world, depending to some extent on our personalities and our values, which can account for significant differences in our perceptions. How we react to what is going on around us and to the interactions we have with others is often determined by our particular way of viewing the world and the behavior patterns we use to get along in it. You can probably get right on track with some patients and yet have difficulty understanding or interviewing others. In this chapter, we describe various characteristics and behavior patterns of patients and demonstrate how you can quickly apply this information to your communications with your patients.

Over the years, psychologists such as Carl Jung and many others have looked at how people's personalities and coping skills vary and what effects this can have on their interactions. Evaluation of personality type has become standard practice in the corporate world during the last two decades, and it's not surprising that personality assessment services are a sizable business for human resource consultants.

A CONVENIENT TOOL FOR UNDERSTANDING OTHERS

For use in the Desmond Medical Communications workshops, I have adapted one particular body of research on what is referred to as the four social styles (Reid and Merrill, 1981). This serves as a practical and convenient tool to help clinicians gain insights into their patients and quickly determine what behaviors a particular patient may prefer and what that person may respond to most positively. This knowledge can affect many aspects of communicating with a patient, from how you listen or explain about medications to how you greet them or say goodbye. In later chapters, we refer to these four social styles, so the more familiar you are with the dominant characteristics of each, the easier it will be for you to apply all the other communication techniques in this book.

THE FOUR SOCIAL STYLES

The four social styles we meet here are the Analytical, the Driving, the Expressive, and the Amiable. Figure 3.1 shows the four social styles laid out in quadrants. The horizontal and vertical lines that intersect to form the quadrants should each be considered a continuum with gradients of the social styles running along them, becoming more pronounced at the extreme ends.

The horizontal line measures degrees of assertiveness, with the most assertive patients on the far right and the least assertive on the far left. Patients anywhere in the right half of the figure are in the two assertive styles: Driving and Expressive. They tend to direct people or tell them what they want.

Those in the left half of the figure (the Analyticals and Amiables) are comfortable with tranquil interactions and dislike overt conflict.

The vertical continuum measures a person's value system, or preference for a particular focus. Task focus increases as we go up. Driving and

Figure 3.1. The Four Basic Social Styles of Patients

Task Focus: Doing and thinking
- Less responsive
- Controls emotions

Analytical Patient	Driving Patient
Task-oriented	Task-oriented
Prefers to work alone	Likes to be in control
Slow response; accuracy important	Rapid response; quick decisions
Likes to organize, solve puzzles	Prefers immediate, direct action
Likes details, precise measuring	Wants bottom-line results ASAP!
Relationships are a lower priority	Not tactful in relationships
Past-oriented; likes tradition	Present- or future-oriented
Dislikes change; prefers stability	Seeks to manage change
Avoids conflict	More authoritarian under stress
Amiable Patient	**Expressive Patient**
Relationship-oriented	Relationship-oriented
Likes to be member of a group	Likes to stand out in a group
Slower response; wants to please	Rapid, unique response; impulsive
Loyal, supportive, empathic	Verbal, humorous, creative
Senses others' needs and concerns	Dislikes dullness or routine
Good at one-on-one relationship	Motivating and persuasive
Focus on the present	Future focus, visionary
Avoids change; prefers the familiar	Enjoys change; sees opportunity
Avoids conflict	Uses personal attack in conflict

Less Assertive — *More Assertive*

Relationship Focus: Relating and feeling
- More responsive
- Emotes

Source: Adapted from Reid and Merrill (1981).

Analytical patients are somewhere in the upper half of the figure. They tend to be involved and interested in what has to be done, the task at hand, with less focus placed on relationships.

Toward the bottom end of the vertical continuum the preference is for relating to others. A priority for these types, the Amiable patients and Expressive patients, is warm, personal interaction. They are comfortable expressing their feelings and are often guided by them. They also have greater facility for expressing emotions (love, sorrow, and the like).

Again, these axis lines are continua, marking off large areas character-ized by particular behavior patterns and attitudes (some of which are spelled out in Figure 3.1). A person may have a few but not all of the traits of a particular quadrant or social style. Some patients, therefore, can be full-on Driving types, having most of the traits of this style, whereas others might be "sort of" Driving and have only some of the traits in the Driving style and some in another.

No Easy Labels

Before we go further, we must make one important caveat. This tool is not in-tended as a means of totally defining a particular person, or for oversimplified labeling of patients or anyone else. We are all far too complex to fit neatly into one of the four distinct quadrants in the figure. We have observed that many people (if not most) operate in all four social styles at various times through-out the day. However, researchers tell us that people tend to have one domi-nant style, usually the quadrant they are most comfortable in and to which they retreat if they are under stress (Reid and Merrill, 1981). We think you'll find that as you work with this tool, it becomes progressively easier to use.

Advantages for Communicating

One specific benefit of tuning into your patients' social styles is that you can react to their behaviors in a way that is easier on you emotionally. A patient's aggressive behavior, for example, may be attributed to social style rather than being interpreted as a direct attack against you. What appears to be rude or aloof behavior in another patient may be due, in large part, to how a person with that social style typically reacts under stress.

When we ask physicians and other clinicians who have previously par-ticipated in the Desmond Medical Communications workshops "What did you get out of the class that was especially useful?" many respond as did one family physician recently: "I try to work with a patient's style now, be more sensitive to it, and that usually helps. But I also don't get on myself as much when I don't seem to be on track with a certain person. I realize that we have different personalities, and that's OK."

Why This Approach?

There are other personality instruments that are more complex and comprehensive, notably the Myers-Briggs Type Indicator (MBTI), which has sixteen distinct descriptions of personality type (Myers and Briggs, 1990). But we have found that the tool presented in Figure 3.1, with only four social styles, is easier to understand and more convenient to use. Again, it is introduced here primarily for quickly gauging the general parameters of a patient's communication preferences. What is a particular patient likely to react to, positively or negatively? How can you present information in such a way that it is likely to be heard and remembered by that patient?

This Is Useful for All Your Relationships

You may be able to apply some of these insights on social styles and the related techniques for using them to a variety of situations in both your professional and your personal life—for example, when dealing with a colleague, a friend, your spouse, or other family members. You will have new skills for reducing conflict and understanding their behaviors.

No Style Is Better Than Another

What is particularly comforting in this approach is that it is not judgmental. There is no right or wrong social style—none is better than any other. Certain styles may be better suited to particular career paths than others, but no social style is inherently superior to another. Each has its own advantages and disadvantages.

Clues to Determining Your Patient's Social Style

When you first meet a new patient, what are the clues that help you determine his or her social style? In describing the four styles, we include a subsection entitled "How to Spot Them." This lists some of the behaviors particular to that style that can tip you off as to the patient's probable communication preferences, at least to some extent.

You may need to refer back to this section frequently as you begin using this tool, but soon you will find you can pick up clues quickly on your own. For example, patients who are relaters (Amiable or Expressive patients) tend to use more affect generally than Analytical and Driving patients. They are likely to react to what you say with head nodding and facial expressions.

Now let's look at the four social styles in terms of how they might respond to you and to the health care situation in general.

DRIVING PATIENTS

Driving patients generally like to control situations and other people. They focus on the task at hand and are often somewhat authoritarian in their approach to dealing with others.

Preferences

Driving patients tend to take charge of situations and people. If someone must take over, Driving patients are there, running things, preferably their way. They like speed, efficiency, and a no-nonsense approach (which sometimes translates as "Don't bother me with details and a lot of emotional stuff!"). They are able to make fast decisions and like immediate, direct action that gets fast, solid results. Conversations often revolve around projects they are doing or what they have done recently. These are action people.

Time Orientation

Driving patients tend to be focused on the present and, to a lesser extent, the future. They are not particularly interested in what has happened in the past or in the traditional way of doing things. But they are definitely interested in the state of things right now and in the near future. They want things done today—for a better tomorrow. Driving patients are usually not put off by change; rather, they try to figure out how to manage it. They typically like to decide quickly what to do and get on with it. Details and delays can irritate them.

Relationships

Although relationships are important to Driving patients, one of the traits of this social style is that they are often not careful about how they relate to others. They often forget to edit their words before they say them, which can put a big dent in their relationships. Instead, they tend to lay things on the line and just blurt it out. They may not be skilled at couching their message in gentle terms, nor take the time to figure out how to say things sensitively. Occasionally, these patients may seem somewhat rude, abrupt, or even demanding. You are likely to pick up this assertiveness in a Driving patient right from the start, at your first encounter.

I have observed that patients who have the tendencies of this style tend to prefer clinicians who share some of their traits. They seem to respect each other's apparent strength: the strong, fast, self-assured voice; the large body gestures; the let's-move-forward attitude; and the preference for direct action. With many Driving patients, it may seem as if they are always scanning every human interaction to see what kind of mettle they're dealing with—as if they are taking one's measure: *Where's the backbone here? How far can I push? Where are the limits?* They may do this at the conscious or the unconscious level. No doubt you have dealt with people who have some of these traits.

How to Spot Them

Driving patients tend to speak rapidly, in short, clipped sentences. They use few words, but those they use are meaningful, targeted, and important. Their voices may be louder than others, and (like the Analytical patients we meet in the next section) their voices tend to have fewer intonations.

Driving patients' gestures are often big, firm, and very definite. The palms are generally closed, but they may use pointing gestures. They often take up space, spreading out as they talk—resting an elbow on the corner of the desk; feet apart; and handbags, books, or briefcases spread out nearby. When they want to make a point, they usually do it strongly and assertively, leaning forward, using direct eye contact and a firm, fast, strong delivery.

Under Stress

Driving patients tend to respond decisively in a crisis. This is one of their strengths and also one of their weaknesses. They tend to become more authoritarian and more task-oriented when they are stressed. They may start barking orders: "I do *not* want to be kept waiting like this! My appointment was for two o'clock. It's two now. I insist on being seen immediately!" Or in another scenario, "I've had enough of your 'Let's-try-this—let's-try-that' stuff. Make up your mind, and let's get something that *works!* I'm sick of this pain. If you can't fix it, I'll find someone who can!"

It can be decidedly tense dealing with patients who have a predominantly Driving style, especially if you have a milder social style and dislike conflict. If conflict does occur, however, use the technique we describe in the later subsection titled "Be Prepared to Deal with a Frontal Attack" (in the section on Expressives). If the conflict occurs because you were running late and kept the patient waiting long after the appointment time, we strongly suggest making some cost adjustment for that visit, since patients with this social style are often attracted to financial rewards.

How to Get on Track with Them

If your style is quite different, it often helps to use some of the characteristics of the Driving patient's own style as you interact. Try to speak a little more rapidly, with a stronger, slightly louder voice, lower in your vocal range. Lean forward slightly, avoid holding your upper arms close to your body, and use somewhat bigger gestures. If you use this kind of body language and vocal quality, your Driving patients are likely to take you seriously and be respectful and attentive.

Avoid using the word *feel* with this social style; instead, use the word *think. Think* is also a better word to use with Analytical patients, since they also tend to focus on thinking more than on feeling and will probably relate better to this word.

Since Driving patients are strongly attracted to moving forward efficiently, winning the race, and achieving good results, these are the very words and metaphors they like to use in their own language: *results, achieve, win, efficient, bottom line, move on, get it done, deal with it,* and so forth. They also like to hear others talk this way and are likely to respond positively when they hear this kind of "doing" or "controlling" language.

Tips for Working with the Driving Patient

Be Punctual. Swiftness is important to these people. They don't like to take time away from work or other responsibilities, so don't keep them waiting. They are particularly irritated by delays, and if they have to wait longer than expected when they come to see you, you will probably hear about it. It's often a good idea to schedule the Driving patient for the first office visit of the morning or the first appointment of the afternoon, whenever you are least likely to be running late.

Stick to the Facts. Driving patients often prefer the clinician who spares the small talk and warm fuzzies and gets down to business. Some opening small talk is still our recommendation, as well as acknowledgment of their psychosocial concerns (if they reveal them). Try to keep your responses fairly brief, however, and certainly not emotionally cloying in any way. Heavy doses of sympathy are not generally welcome with this social style; say nothing that smacks of "Awww, poor you."

Give Them Choices. Having control is important to Driving patients. They may want to make at least some of the decisions about their health care options, even minor ones, to retain some sense of control over their situation. For instance, if a Driving patient has hypertension and requires medication, you could explain the side effects of the various appropriate medications and let the patient have a voice in choosing which medication he or she prefers.

Be Brief. Unless they ask for or seem to want a lengthy, detailed explanation, you may find that Driving patients prefer a concise explanation that just covers the key points. Detailed explanations (perhaps with references to historic developments of various treatment modalities) are likely to go over better with your Analytical patients.

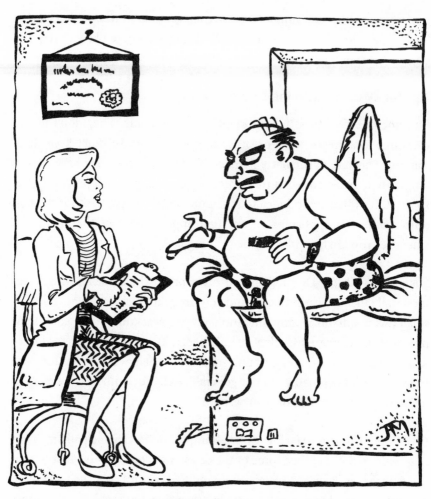

"Doc, it's no use telling me to stop smoking,
drinking, overeating. . . . How I *get* my problems is my
business. . . . Getting rid of them is *your* business!"

Source: Cartoon by James A. Moseley. Copyright 1996 Desmond Medical Communications.

Driving patients usually want to know the essentials, the critical elements, and the bottom line. People like this are often very successful in business, and they're used to dealing with their management team this way. When they come to you for your expertise, they want you to give them good, solid advice, preferably quickly and succinctly, as to the best way to get the bottom-line results you both want for their particular situation.

ANALYTICAL PATIENTS

Analytical patients are often slow, methodical, and precise in examining all of the issues. In general, they are more logical and less emotional than the general population in their overall view of the world. Like Driving patients, they also tend to be task-oriented, but they are less assertive and in some cases they may even be a bit passive.

Preferences

Patients who have traits of this style usually like information: reports, data, statistics, graphs, measurements, and numbers. Rules and standards are important. They like to adhere to them and wish that others would do the same. They enjoy solving puzzles and are quite good at it.

The old saying "A place for everything and everything in its place" was surely coined by an Analytical somewhere. They like their surroundings kept neat and orderly, with everything in its assigned place.

Analytical patients usually are not comfortable standing out in a crowd or being in the spotlight; they generally don't like having attention called to themselves. They tend to be less outgoing and somewhat more introverted than those influenced by the other three social styles.

Time Orientation

Because people with this social style tend to focus on the past and cherish their routines and traditions, change can be very troublesome for them. It disrupts the orderliness they prefer, and it interferes with established ways of doing things. They can be quite upset by changes, especially those that are sudden or unannounced.

Relationships

Analytical patients don't seem to need the company of other people as much as those in the other three quadrants do. They often like to work alone, or with another Analytical. (If two Analyticals work together, they probably do so in separate rooms—or even separate states, using e-mail.)

Patients with Analytical traits may put considerable effort into the task they have to do, letting their personal relationships take a back seat. But they bring a great deal of effort to gathering information and thoroughly examining all aspects of their health problems—and they are likely to expect you to do the same.

These patients may surf the Internet and download and bring in the latest health care information (correct or incorrect) at the time of their visit. They may be a bit shy at times, which others may read as being somewhat aloof. This common perception of coolness is also due to their tendency to concentrate fully on what they are hearing or reading. As with Driving patients, Analyticals tend to direct their primary energy to the task. They like thinking about things, whereas "feeling about things" may not occur as often.

How to Spot Them

Analytical patients generally speak slowly, often in a monotone. They may pause frequently to find the most accurate word to precisely express their meaning. Their affect tends to be lower than any of the other three social styles. As you speak to them, you may notice they react less and maintain a fairly expressionless face. Their eye contact is indirect; they often focus on objects or on written information as they talk.

These patients use few gestures, and those they use are contained (for example, elbows are often held close to the body). They tend to sit in a fairly erect position or lean back, but they are not likely to lean forward, and they generally don't spread out or gesture vigorously as they interact with others.

Communicating with Today's Patient

Listen to what they talk about and the terms in which they describe their symptoms. Analytical patients generally talk about facts and data and the task to be accomplished. Mention of their feelings and fears, friends, and family may not come up much in their conversation.

Your Analytical patients may include engineers, mathematicians, accountants, librarians, or people who handle details, numbers, and precise measurements. Analytical personalities are often drawn to professions of this kind.

Under Stress

If there is conflict or stress, Analytical patients tend to go quietly away, to withdraw and involve themselves in something that occupies their minds. They may be right there in the room with you, but they can "pull down the shade," in effect, and simply not be available. They may retreat behind a newspaper or become absorbed in a book, or they may actually drift out the door and leave (not slamming the door, though; that is more the style of Driving or Expressive patients).

Because Analytical patients tend to avoid conflict, they may just disappear from your practice when they are dissatisfied, but you will probably never know why or what it was about. They dislike open complaining or confrontation, tending instead to just avoid an unpleasant situation. People in this quadrant of Figure 3.1 tend to express their anger covertly rather than overtly. (Amiable patients, a style we meet shortly, are also conflict-averse, but they handle it differently.)

How to Get on Track with Them

Use few facial expressions and almost no gestures. Sit up or lean back, but sit a little farther away from these patients than you might with others. Analytical patients, and sometimes Driving patients, tend to prefer appreciably greater "social distance" than do those with the other two social styles. With most people, acceptable social distance (how close they want to be to others) is between two and four feet. With Analytical patients, it may be somewhat further away.

If you lean forward too much as you talk with Analytical patients, they may back away slightly or even move the chair back to maintain their need for greater social distance. Don't take this personally, since they probably react this way to others who come too close to them physically.

Keep your voice even and modulated as you talk with them, and use few intonations. If you normally speak rapidly, try to slow down.

An Analytical patient's slow and logical responses can be irritating to Driving or Expressive types. You have probably seen this in couples who have distinctly different social styles. While the husband, with traits of the Analytical patient, is trying to tell you his symptoms, verrry slowly and in precise detail, his Driving or Expressive wife may blurt out, "Just *say* it, Jack! The doctor doesn't have all day!" or she may move in and do the talking for him.

People who have very different styles can get on each other's nerves; yet it's surprising how often people with opposite social styles, such as Driving and Amiable or Analytical and Expressive are marriage partners or life partners. Analytical patients may have particular difficulty relating to those with the social style we meet next, the Expressive patient, whose tendency for big and bold statements and behaviors may be uncomfortable for Analyticals. They may see this behavior as too emotional and showy—not precise, thoughtful, and scientific, which they prefer.

A few years back, a popular female comic described her obviously Analytical father: "You wanna know what drives my father ab-so-lutely crazy? You take a road map and unfold it—all the way out. Then instead of folding it exactly, precisely the way it was, you crunch it all up, fast, into a big, messy ball. Drives him crazy."

Tips for Working with Analytical Patients

Prepare an Agenda. Analytical patients like to have an agenda in advance, an overview of what the steps are along the way, whether it's a complex treatment plan or just a routine office visit. We recommend an orientation for all your patients early in the visit, giving them a general overview of how you'll proceed, but it's especially important to provide

Communicating with Today's Patient

such an informal agenda for your Analytical patients. For instance, they may appreciate a statement such as "After we talk awhile about the symptoms you've been having, I'll examine you, and then we can discuss a treatment approach for you."

Give Them a Map and a Timetable. Analytical patients also want to know exactly where they go to get their tests or medications. As we point out in Chapter Six on explanations, they like maps and specific written instructions as to where they go for their tests and what they are to do after that. These patients are also likely to want to know how long it will take to receive the results of the lab tests, x-rays, ultrasounds, and so forth, since they put emphasis on precision and the linear order of events. Once you discuss how long it takes to get the results back, make certain you carry through and notify them of these studies in a timely manner. It might be best to give a broader range of time: "within a week" rather than "by next Tuesday or Wednesday" or "in about two days." Because of their precision, Analytical patients may hold you to any specific dates you mention.

Provide Details. This type of patient usually likes detailed explanations that include plenty of numbers, percentages, and even charts and graphs. For example, if you can download from your office computer the extrapolated growth rates of your pediatric patient for an Analytical parent, it will be especially well received.

Analytical patients want you to be as accurate, logical, and precise as they are. They probably read every detail on the bills they receive from you as well as the small print on their health plan contract. They are even likely to read the small-print inserts in medications!

Clearly, the cartoon on the next page shows an Analytical clinician giving directions. If the driver is also an Analytical, she may even understand what he is saying! If she's not, she's still lost—and befuddled as well.

Be Neat and Clean. Because Analytical patients prefer neatness and organization, a messy office or bulletin board with pictures and cartoons

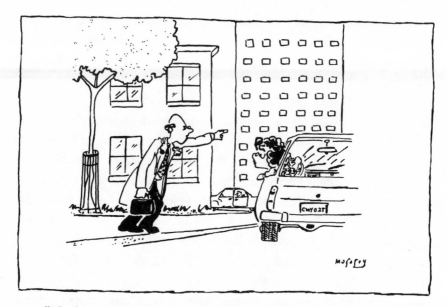

"The hospital? Sure. . . . proceed to the first dextral diverticulum,
deviate ipsilaterally, subtend the proximal stop sign,
and you can't miss it."

Source: Cartoon by James A. Moseley. Copyright 1996 Desmond Medical Communications.

hanging at odd angles or piled on top of one another is likely to irritate them.

Because of their focus on the past and their preference for longstanding tradition, they are often conservative in their tastes and preferences. They may bristle at a clinician who is dressed too informally or "inappropriately." For more specifics on this, see Chapter Ten, "Shining Up Your Professional Image."

Provide Sufficient Resources. Patients with this social style may not want to join a support group for their medical condition, preferring instead to read information you give them concerning their health problem or attend your clinic's lectures on the topic. Nevertheless, let them know of support groups so that they can decide whether to attend.

Analytical patients often defer making decisions about surgery or other procedures until they absorb sufficient information on the topic to make a "correct" decision. If you tell this type of patient "I strongly recommend that you have your gallbladder removed as soon as possible. Shall we decide on a time to schedule the surgery?" The Analytical patient's response may well be: " I'm not sure about setting a date just yet. Do you have any information I can read about this surgery?" The problem one often encounters is that Analyticals can defer too long because they never have quite enough data. They may need a bit of nudging. It can often take two or more visits or telephone calls before they come to a decision of any sort.

Present Both Sides of the Issue. The pros and cons, the advantages and the disadvantages of a particular approach are important to the Analytical patient, who may, for example, ask about the cost-benefit ratios of a procedure or the statistics on outcomes of a surgical intervention. It can often be helpful to sit down with an Analytical patient, fold a piece of paper in half, and jot down the two sides of the issue. With this approach, the patient can see it clearly laid out and can take it home for further consideration.

Be Considerate of Information That the Patient Brings In. As we mentioned, Analytical patients may come in with information they have downloaded from the Internet on the latest procedures or medications. Or they may have cut out an article from a newspaper or journal. Bringing in medical information from the media—radio, television, electronic and print media—certainly isn't restricted to patients with this social style; other types of patients may do so as well. But since Analyticals are especially keen on data, these people are most likely to bring printed information to their medical visits.

Many physicians in our workshops tell us they are put off when patients come in waving articles they have read or downloaded. Their feeling is, "Hey, am I the doctor here or not?" Our suggestion is that since this is happening with ever greater frequency (from what we can tell), you might as well deal with it in a way that leaves everybody smiling. Rather than being defensive, feeling your role as the authority is being undermined, go with their style. Use it to your benefit.

Here is a three-step approach for dealing with situations like this.

First, acknowledge your patients' active role and their interest in their own health care.

Second, be sure to thank them for contributing information. It might be new information you haven't seen yet (especially if it's freshly downloaded) and that might be interesting and useful. Patients bring these articles in with the expectation, in most cases, that you will appreciate their contribution. This is the behavior of actively involved patients, accepting more responsibility for their own health care and assuming more of a partnership role with you—exactly what is needed for greater patient compliance. Encourage this attitude with a gracious "thank you" at least. Lanny always thanks his patients for gathering information. He adds that even though some of the articles they bring in may have incorrect information, he sees this as an opportunity to educate patients about what is appropriate.

Third, show respect for the data. For example, tell them you will read it over at your first opportunity. ("Reading over" is not quite the same as reading word-for-word, which your busy schedule may not allow.)

Avoid taking a few seconds right then to just skim down the information quickly, finding some reason to discount it; doing so definitely pushes the patient's buttons. You can assume they have read it thoroughly and think it has merit. If you don't think it does, we suggest you at least give them some of the pros as well as the cons of the article, or better yet defer your reaction until later, by putting it with the chart and telling them you'll read it over soon. Again, be sure to acknowledge their interest in learning more about their own health issues.

If you say you'll look at the information, be sure you follow up on it. Jot down a note, perhaps with the patient's chart, to discuss it on the next visit. They are likely to remember to bring it up and will be disappointed if you haven't at least become familiar with the material.

Keep in mind that Analytical patients put a high priority on data. Whatever they bring in to you needs to be respected, even if you don't agree with the information entirely. At least recognize it as an intended contribution to the health care puzzle you are both trying to figure out. This approach is also useful with other patients, since, as we mentioned, it's not only your Analytical patients who will bring in articles or who fax or e-mail this kind of update to you. And by the way, if this hasn't happened to you yet, it will.

AMIABLE PATIENTS

Amiable people are often surrounded by their friends and family. Amiable patients are very good relaters who respond and react based on their feelings much of the time. They like to make others happy and comfortable, even at a cost to themselves. They tend to avoid conflict or any action that might distress others—especially someone they care for.

Preferences

Amiable patients tend to prefer one-on-one interactions, but they also enjoy being with groups of friends. In a group, they don't particularly want to be the leader or to stand out in any way. They just like being there, as a solid member of the group, loved and appreciated. They are usually the ones who bring the holiday treats into your office or clinic so the staff can all enjoy the holiday together.

Time Orientation

Amiable patients often talk and move unhurriedly and usually prefer a warm, chatty conversation over getting down to business and working on the task at hand. Their major time focus is " right now," especially if they are doing something enjoyable with friends and loved ones.

Amiable patients can have a difficult time with change; in some cases they even go through a kind of grieving process when major changes occur to them or their loved ones.

Relationships

Because Amiable patients put a priority on relationships, they seem to have a kind of "sensitivity database" they can tap into to understand the feelings and motivations of others. They often have excellent intuition about people. It's a source of information that those who are more analytical do not seem to have.

How to Spot Them

Amiable patients usually have very responsive facial expressions and head movements, smiling and nodding as you talk to them. They are likely to be somewhat slow in speaking, and their responses to your questions may be slow too. They may have some inflection in their voices but none as dramatic as with the Expressive patient, whom we meet next. They tend to make few statements, but they particularly like to talk about people who are emotionally important to them, such as friends and family members. Their conversation with you may go something like this: "Well, my son's wife said she thought . . ." or "My next door neighbor was over yesterday with his wife . . . they were just back from their trip to France and wanted to tell us all about it and anyway, they were saying that they had met a man on their trip who also had dizziness like mine and he had been trying. . . ."

Amiable patients often sit in a relaxed position, leaning back. Their gestures use mainly the lower arm and are often primarily small or circular movements of the hands. They tend to sit or stand in a contained way, arms and elbows close to the body, in contrast to the spreading out of the more assertive personalities of the Driving and Expressive patients. Like the Analytical patients, who are also on the less assertive side of Figure 3.1, the Amiable patients tend to ask more than tell. Listen to their language: "Well, if it's OK with you" or "Let me just ask you. . . ."

Under Stress

Amiable patients may cry when under stress, either outwardly or inwardly. Crying outwardly is usually done as a gentle, soft, emotional response, not

Communicating with Today's Patient

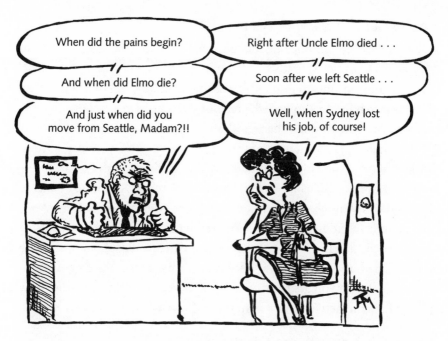

Source: Cartoon by James A. Moseley. Copyright 1996 Desmond Medical Communications.

characterized by a lot of noise or wailing (as might be the case with the Expressive patient). Long-term "inward crying," of course, may show up in symptoms.

A notable exception to this, however, is when Amiable patients stuff their displeasure, which they tend to do. Their angry feelings then build up over time and suddenly surface all at once in a dramatic outburst. One small incident can unleash this collected anger, leaving the person who is the recipient of the outburst perplexed and wondering, "What did I do or say to cause that kind of explosion?" It's often not that single incident, but rather all the bottled-up anger over similar situations in the past that finally bursts out when ignited by a small but related incident.

Lanny adds a word of caution: occasionally these patients, being highly relational, can become too dependent on the physician, which can cause problems.

How to Get on Track with Them

If they are in their schmoozing mode ("Oh, let me tell you about my trip to Hawaii last week. Well, first we . . ."), you should listen for a while at least, giving them your full attention. Because the main function of talk for these patients is to build or reinforce the relationship, this is in part how they feel connected to you, through sharing what is important to them.

If you are a task-oriented or assertive type yourself, you may have to work at actually slowing down and reacting to them, with facial expressions and interjected acknowledgments as they speak. A minute or two of this kind of listening and attention seems like twice the time to an Amiable patient (although it may seem like quadruple the time to you!). It works much the same way with Expressive patients. People in both these relating quadrants prefer facial affect and verbal acknowledgments from you—signals that you are relating to them in a caring, empathic way. They require this interactivity more than the two task-focused styles do.

Tips for Working with Amiable Patients

Make It Safe to Talk About Emotional Issues. Because Amiable patients are very good at sensing the needs and concerns of others, they hope you will do the same for them. If they sense that they can talk with you about their psychosocial issues, which may be associated with their somatic concerns, they are likely to stay with you for the long run. They are generally loyal and supportive if you establish a caring relationship with them, one in which they feel safe talking about their emotional concerns as well as their physical difficulties.

Favor the word *feel* instead of *think* as you talk with your Amiable (and Expressive) patients: "How do you feel about that?" rather than "What do you think about that?" It's helpful to bring out in the open what feelings they have about your recommendations. As we mentioned, if they are unhappy or angry about something you have done or not done, Amiable patients usually don't tell you right to your face. To avoid conflict, they are likely to smile and cover up their discomfort or dissatisfaction. You may hear about it later, however, when an irate family member—

often a more assertive spouse or friend—champions their cause and lodges a complaint.

Dig for the Real Concern. Try to get Amiable patients to anticipate possible hurdles they may face in adhering to the treatment plan. Such prompting for their realistic assessment is important, since they may not come right out and tell you their fears or concerns. These patients are not apt to be forthright, not likely to tell you, for instance, "I can't possibly take time off work to do what you're telling me to do" or "How can I stick to a low-fat diet when my husband wants me to cook his favorite traditional dishes, which are high in fat?" Yet you do need to anticipate such problems, so that you can try to find some solutions together before the patient leaves. Ask open-ended questions: "How will this affect your daily schedule?" or "How do you sense your family will react to your new low-fat diet?" This kind of open-ended question is especially important with Amiable patients and can affect their adherence.

It may be difficult to get the real presenting complaint from your Amiable patients. They may not tell you straight out what they are really concerned about. Because Amiable patients are people pleasers, if they have a health problem they feel is shameful or revolting in any way, they may withhold it. Because of their emotion-based behaviors, these are often the patients with a hidden agenda. They may cover up what they are really afraid of with a smile or demurral of some sort, and let the secret out only after they realize that the visit has come to an end. "Oh, by the way" happens frequently with patients who have this social style.

Since long-term relationships are important to Amiable patients, it can be very difficult for them if they have to switch from a cherished physician to a new one when they move or change health plans. You might begin your first interaction with them by saying, "I'm very pleased to have you as my patient, (use the patient's name). I know I can never replace Dr. (use that clinician's name). But I'll give you my complete attention when you come to see me, and I hope that as time goes on you'll feel comfortable and well taken care of—as I know you did with her." This kind of introduction, or some variation of it, is a good way to begin your relationship with any new patient, of course, but it is particularly effective with Amiable patients—and Expressive patients.

EXPRESSIVE PATIENTS

Expressive patients also enjoy relating to others. They love to talk and enjoy being with other people, especially if they can be center stage or up in front of them in some way. They tend to be very outgoing and playful, and they like to involve other people in their activities.

Preferences

Expressive patients thrive on recognition, uniqueness, and status. What they don't like is anything routine, dull, or standardized. They love variety, creativity, and spontaneity and are quickly bored with the commonplace or routine.

Expressive patients can often be excitable and impulsive. If you ask them a question, you probably won't get a standard answer. It will likely be something unique, clever, or funny.

Time Orientation

Expressive patients do have one particular quality that is very important in today's world. Because they tend to be oriented toward the future, they often have an uncanny ability to sense what the future holds and are frequently somewhat visionary. They can often see things coming, such as new trends, before others can. These patients rather enjoy change and like the challenge of coming up with creative solutions for dealing with it. Because of this ability and their enjoyment of the new and the novel, Expressives tend to be highly innovative.

Relationships

Expressive patients like to be part of a group (as do Amiable patients), but they like to be an outstanding member in some way. They enjoy being in the spotlight. They are proud of any titles they might have, especially ones that give them status and prestige, such as colonel, judge, or dean. Be sure to use Expressive patients' names—their last name and any title they may have. Also, they like to have you acknowledge any recent achievement or any publicity they may have received.

How to Spot Them

Expressive patients generally use fast speech and a loud voice with lots of inflection and dramatic variety. They tend to make statements, particularly about their many views on an assortment of topics. They tend to use lots of affect, expressed in strong, fast gestures and large, dynamic movements. Many wear an assortment of rings and other jewelry, and they often like bright, optimistic colors. They like to be noticed! Because they are assertive, they often lean forward to make a point and use direct eye contact as they talk about their symptoms, their opinions, and even their friends and family.

Humor is often part of the mix. Playful and fun loving, these break-the-rules patients can brighten your day, leaving you charged up and amused.

Expressive patients may want the latest breakthrough procedures. Keep in mind that if it's new and in the news, that will make it more attractive to Expressive patients. They may agree to have surgery or some other test or intervention with firm conviction, even setting the date during the visit. But later, after they get home (and talk to their Analytical friends or spouses), they may think better of it, at which time the plans for the intervention or test may be canceled.

Under Stress

This assertive personality becomes very vocal under stress, using big gestures and often a loud voice. Because Expressives are also used to showing their emotions when under stress, they sometimes resort to an in-your-face, highly volatile, personal attack.

They are similar to the Driving patients in that they usually tell you their reactions straight out. However, Expressive patients are likely to tell you overtly how they *feel* about a situation, whereas Driving patients are more apt to tell you overtly what they *think* about it. Since people with Expressive and Driving styles are assertive types, their reactions are big, strong, and often unsettling for those clinicians who dislike conflict and have a somewhat gentle manner.

How to Get on Track with Them

If you don't have a particularly keen sense of humor, be ready at least to laugh when these patients toss off an amusing quip or say something funny, even a full-blown joke. Laughing with them—in the right places— is very important in building rapport.

If your style tends to be unhurried and not particularly assertive, talk a little faster than usual and use a slightly bigger voice with more volume than you ordinarily use. Try to increase inflections and emphasis in your voice as you speak with them. Use plenty of facial affect and gestures, and lean forward as you talk, keeping your shoulders oriented toward them. Expressive patients are likely to want assurance that they have your full attention and that you recognize them as being the unique individuals they are.

Tips for Working with Expressive Patients

Address Patients Using Proper Names and Titles. Because they like to stand out in a crowd, and because they enjoy their own uniqueness, Expressive patients definitely do not want to be lumped with everyone else. They expect you to address them by name and title, and they may be particularly put off if you don't. None of your patients will be as put off as the Expressive patient in this cartoon, we hope, but you can expect to hear— loud and clear—from your dissatisfied Expressive patients.

If you work in a specialty involving care of children, be sure you don't address the parents or refer to them as "Mother" or "Dad." Such generic labeling might irritate or insult them even if they overhear you talking to someone else on the telephone, for example. ("Hi, Jean, Mother is here asking if we have extra blank shot records for her baby. Call me back, will you?") Expressive patients are also particularly sensitive about your using

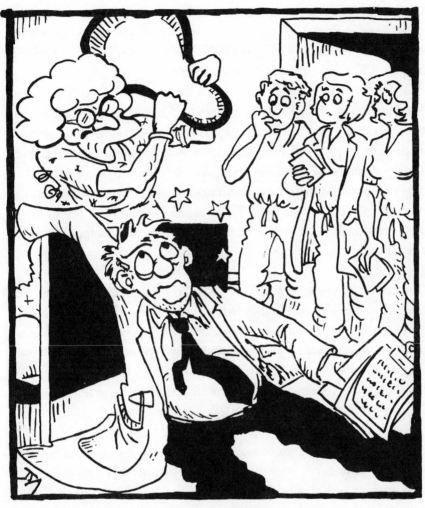

" 'Eighty-one-year-old widowed Caucasian female' nothing,
you rapscallion! My name is Eunice Bascomb,
and from now on I want to hear you say it!"

Source: Cartoon by James A. Moseley. Copyright 1996 Desmond Medical Communications.

the third person singular in referring to them. ("Get his charts," "Find her x-rays," and so forth.) This preference for being recognized as a unique individual is true for all your patients, but it deserves special mention here because it is so important to Expressive patients.

Remind Patients About the Appointment. Since Expressive patients tend to underestimate how much time a particular task or event will take, such as the trip to your office or clinic, they may be late for appointments. Their own personal schedules are often overbooked because of this tendency to underestimate time requirements. With Expressive patients, it might be particularly advisable for someone in the front office to send a postcard or make a telephone call a few days prior to their appointment as a reminder.

Use Visuals. Expressive patients like a show and often appreciate your using plastic models or hand-drawn pictures of the areas of the body affected by their type of illness. Slide shows, videos, and group lectures on their health issues are often appreciated as well. Word pictures and figures of speech can also be especially effective in helping these patients understand what you are explaining to them. For more on these techniques, see Chapter Six.

Help Patients Establish Routines. If they have to do something the same way, at the same time, every day, Expressive patients may have some difficulty sticking with it, since they are easily bored with routine and sameness. If they have to take a certain regimen of medication throughout the week, giving this patient a compartmentalized plastic pill container might be especially helpful; or you might want to prescribe a medication administered only once a day. Talk it over with the patient, as appropriate.

If the patient comes to medical appointments with a relative, that relative might be willing to check the prescribed regimen along with the patient. Handle this delicately so that you don't insult the patient or encourage dependence on the other person. Broaching the idea to the patient and the relative can be done with a gentle suggestion: "Sometimes it's nice to have someone else help you keep track of the medications" or "count the repetitions of knee raises." Finish with, "How do you feel about that?" Pause and await a response.

Be Wary of Possible Manipulation. These patients can also be challenging to deal with, since they may be somewhat manipulative. Some Expressive patients use their keen verbal abilities and their charm to wheedle what they want out of people. (Since it works with other people, it just might work with you too.) Phrases such as "You're the only one who really understands me" are not unusual from manipulative patients who want something that may not be indicated.

If this happens, use *I* messages (such as, "I feel uncomfortable giving you this because it can have some very negative long-term effects; I prefer ...."), then tell them your preference, adding a benefit message (for example, "Because your long-term good health is my number one concern ...."). You might finish the sentence with the patient's name. Lean forward as you say all of this, and be sure you look the patient in the eye and sound sincere. Your appearance should be caring, concerned, and positive, but your body language and tone of voice should match the Expressive patient's assertiveness.

Be Prepared to Deal with a Frontal Attack. Because they are assertive as well as emotional, Expressive patients are likely to let you and everyone else know when they are dissatisfied or angry with their care. They may do this in the form of a verbal, personal attack ("You didn't even have the decency to ..." or "How could you ...?"). There is very little need to prompt or probe for feelings with this social style! They usually come right out and tell you or someone on your staff—as Eunice Bascomb in the earlier cartoon did.

If they do express their anger, acknowledge this at once (assuming it is a relatively minor irritation and not a malpractice issue) by saying, for example, "I'm sorry you were inconvenienced, and I can understand why you'd be upset about having to wait thirty minutes to see me today." Then you can add your explanation or your position on the issue. But always acknowledge their emotional response first, then give your rational or logical explanation after that. If you try to deal with the rational component of the situation before dealing with the emotion, the patient is likely to either not hear you or not respond positively to your explanation.

As we mentioned earlier in this chapter, a technique that often works in this situation (the patient had to wait well beyond the appointment time to see you) is to offer to adjust the cost of that visit, give the patient a voucher for some gift or benefit, or refund the copayment for that day. This is effective for defusing other angry patients, too, not just Expressive and Driving patients. A ten- or twenty-dollar copayment is small compared with the cost of a complaint or a lost patient, as we pointed out in Chapters One and Two. Another defuser is to offer to give the patient the first appointment of the afternoon next time, so there won't be any waiting.

YOUR MOST DIFFICULT PATIENTS

Even though we haven't suggested doing so, by now you have probably placed yourself somewhere on the grid of Figure 3.1. In which quadrant are you most comfortable in your interactions with others? Would other people who know you well agree with that self-identification?

If you have figured out which style is most familiar to you, the one with most of your traits, or the one you retreat to under stress, then your most difficult patients are probably those whose social style lies in the quadrant diagonally across from yours. For example, if you share several of the traits of an Analytical, it may be especially difficult for you to deal with an Expressive patient. If you have many of the qualities of a Driving style, Amiable patients may frequently get on your nerves when they talk too slowly or seem too dependent. You may find yourself thinking, at some level, "Stand up for yourself!" or "Get to the point so we can find a solution here!"

Patients who have social styles distinctly different from yours may get on your nerves, but at least now you know why it's happening. Furthermore, by identifying a patient's probable social style, you can anticipate the areas of potential disconnect or conflict and adjust your communication techniques to avoid such conflict. By being aware of patients' probable responses and preferences, you can react to them in their own manner, using the traits of their social style, which can help them feel comfortable with you as their physician or clinician.

OPPOSITES ATTRACT, IN SOME CASES

Patients may actually prefer a clinician who has a decidedly different social style from their own. An Amiable patient, for example, who is timid and reluctant to move forward with a surgical procedure may prefer a Driving clinician to provide the strength and let's-get-this-done approach that she senses she needs. Or an Expressive patient, concerned about his sudden and unexplained symptoms, may prefer the precise, methodical approach of an Analytical clinician.

BROADENING YOUR COMMUNICATION STYLES

We are sometimes asked in our workshops, "Are you suggesting that I change my personality? That I have to contort myself to try to be like my patients?" Others ask, "Isn't this playacting more than medicine?"

Yes, we are suggesting that you use a few of the behaviors and language preferences of a style other than yours as you interact with a particular patient. No, we are not asking you to be artificial. We prefer to think of it as being more versatile, expanding your repertoire of useful communication approaches, which can improve the care you deliver to patients. You will decide when and how to use these approaches.

In addition, throughout this book we focus on how you can help the patient feel understood and comfortable in talking with you. One way to do that is by using more elements of a style that they can relate to easily— their own. Using these skills doesn't require you to fundamentally change your own personality. Nor does it require you to become manipulative.

Rather, you now have a broader range of communication techniques and greater adaptability to others. After all, it's a reasonable guess that the person whose social style gets on your nerves may not be entirely comfortable with your preferred behaviors either; he or she may feel washed out after having to interact with you and your particular social style.

Adding this versatility to your behavior allows you to speak to people who are different from you in a way that helps them hear you, relate to you positively, and connect with you readily in a therapeutic relationship. We've already discussed all the health care benefits that are associated with that: greater patient adherence, time saving, reduced risk of malpractice, better outcomes, and patient loyalty.

During the coming weeks, if you find yourself thinking *I just can't figure out why I'm not on frequency with this patient,* you might want to look at this chapter again. We are sometimes asked how this relates to what is called the chemistry between two people. When the chemistry (nonsexual) is good between you and a patient, it can be because your preferred social styles—your ways of seeing the world and reaching out to it—are similar.

It's also important to point out that as you work at trying to adjust to someone who has a style different from yours, you may feel a bit tired—physically tired—at least at the beginning. But gradually it becomes easier to slip into this versatility; it even becomes an enjoyable challenge.

This may also be a good opportunity to add more dimensions to your own personality. If you live mostly in your head, easing into a few of the behaviors of your Amiable or Expressive patients might be a good exercise to stretch your own personality. When you tap into your own emotional responses to a patient, it might be just what the doctor ordered, and just what the patient needed.

Conversely, if you base many of your reactions on emotional responses, some practice with a task-oriented, thinking style might give you a broader base of communication skills and allow you to garner greater respect from patients (and staff).

Difficult patients can provide your best learning opportunities. Take these opportunities to stretch your communication skills. Try adjusting to a difficult patient's dominant social style, even though it may be foreign turf to you.

Again, there is no best style, no judgment placed on any particular quadrant in Figure 3.1. To encourage your patients so they listen to you and follow the treatment plan, it can be helpful to speak to them in their own preferred language and from their perspective.

So, to the clinicians who share many of the traits of the Analytical, we say, "You can apply a new awareness of these four social styles and their corresponding traits to interactions with patients to gain more information for an accurate diagnosis and to exponentially increase the potential for patient adherence to the treatment regimen."

To those who share some Driving traits, we say, "Adjust to patients' styles as you talk to them. It gets the job done more efficiently. You get the positive results you want. Your patients don't need to keep coming back because it wasn't done right the first time. They're happy. You're happy."

To the Amiable clinicians, we say, "Being sensitive to how your individual patients view the world and how they may react to what you say strengthens your relationship with them. Even those few patients who are sometimes a little difficult to communicate with will feel more connected and nurtured by you and willing to remain with you as your long-term, loyal patients."

To those of you whose dominant social style is Expressive, we say, "Try it! You'll find it's stimulating to explore social styles and be more simpatico with different kinds of people. Patients will love it! They'll say, 'What a terrific clinician—one of a kind!'"

Speaking in the same personality language as your patients has been the focus of this chapter. But there is also a silent language you speak every day to your patients: body language. Even though it's silent, it can be the loudest thing you say to patients. That's coming up in the next chapter.

CHAPTER 4

Louder Than Words

What Your Body Language
Says to Patients

"Good morning, I'm Dr. Jones," the ophthalmologist announces with his back to the patient as he washes his hands. He then moves directly to his desk and looks down to read the chart as he mumbles in a flat, monotone voice, "Nice to meet you. I see you're interested in contact lenses."

The new patient tells him her concerns about whether contact lenses can help her vision problems, as he continues to read and make notes in the chart. Then he rises without saying a word and begins busily arranging his various ophthalmic medical devices—still with an expressionless face.

Finally, the ophthalmologist faces his new patient and looks her right in the eye—but from the other side of a huge slit lamp sandwiched between them.

When the exam is over, he moves the device out of the way and, to the patient's surprise, focuses on her directly, face to face. She feels that at last she has the physician's personal attention and interest. His words come out very precisely: "The contact lenses and the fitting will cost you two hundred and fifty dollars."

Distant, aloof, and money-grubbing, thinks the patient. *The only time he really looked at me was when he talked money.* She never returns.

Nonverbal communication, which includes both body language and vocal intonation, can transmit feelings and preferences involuntarily—through a sort of "leakage" of attitude. Although you probably wouldn't interact with a patient as this ophthalmologist did, you may not be aware of all the nonverbal messages you're sending each day or how patients are receiving them. The way you stand or sit, your facial expressions and gestures, your personal appearance—all are part of your body language. Since you are constantly sending out these messages each day, it's worth taking some time to consider what they might be saying.

In Chapters One and Two, we talked about the importance of establishing a relationship of trust and the critical role patients' perceptions play in whether they stay with you and accept your medical advice. In this chapter, we look at how profoundly body language influences those objectives.

WHAT COUNTS?

When the ophthalmologist looks down and continues to read the chart as he greets the patient, his words "Nice to meet you" are completely overshadowed by what his body language says: "I'm interested only in the medical data." As much as 55 percent of the message communicated to the patient regarding his attitude and feelings is carried in his body language. The actual words he uses weigh in at only 7 percent. Another 38 percent of his attitude is conveyed by his tone of voice. Since he uses a flat, monotone voice to say, "Nice to meet you," 93 percent of the message transmitted to the patient is more like, "You're just another faceless medical case to me." Albert Mehrabian, professor emeritus at UCLA, determined this breakdown of message components through years of research, conveyed in his scholarly book *Non-Verbal Communication* (1972).

Your body language, even such a small movement as a slight widening of your eyes, can convey quite clearly your level of interest in your patients as you listen to them. Your capacity to empathize with their feelings can be revealed by a mere wrinkling of your forehead as the patient describes

Communicating with Today's Patient

painful symptoms. It requires no extra time to communicate these important messages of caring and interest. Conversely, if you are feeling tired or bored or don't quite believe what your patient is telling you, your body language can just as easily give away your true feelings and send a negative message that the patient quickly picks up.

The extent to which patients dislike negative body language in their clinicians is illustrated in a study conducted by Tony Carr, M.D., associate professor of psychiatry at McMasters University. Forty phobia patients had therapy sessions with a computerized program. They also had sessions with a live therapist. Asked which they preferred, almost 50 percent of the patients said they preferred the computer to the therapist and found the computer much easier to communicate with. "People perceive the computer as being much less authoritarian and judgmental," says Dr. Carr. "It doesn't raise its eyebrows, tap its fingers on the desk or look at its watch" (McAuliffe, 1991, p. 104).

Much of your professional training emphasized *what* you say to patients, and *when*. But *how* you convey information to your patients—through body language and vocal intonation—can outweigh your choice of words by a whopping nine to one!

As the first female television news anchor in New England, I learned, the hard way, many of the skills and techniques that are now part of our Desmond Medical Communications workshops for physicians and other health care professionals. Spending more than fifteen years in broadcast news has taught me a truism in the world of media: the visual always overwhelms the content. It's a new spin on the old adage that it's not what you say but how you say it. The specific relevance to physicians is that whatever your patients see—a downcast or bored expression, a slight tightening of the mouth and jaw, or a smile of pleasure—can overwhelm anything you might be saying, especially if the two don't track.

Ralph Waldo Emerson understood this more than a century ago when he said, "When the eyes say one thing, and the tongue another, a practised man relies on the language of the first" (Emerson, 1941, p. 426). Long before social scientists had measured and quantified body language, Emerson knew intuitively that when facial expressions or other body language don't agree with the words that are being spoken, we all believe the former. We go instinctively with the visual message, believing what we see and read in the body language more than the actual words spoken. That's why this chapter is titled "Louder Than Words."

Studies indicate that physicians who are able to express their emotions through body language tend to receive higher ratings from patients on the art of care, as distinguished from the technical quality of care (DiMatteo, Hays, and Prince, 1986). Body language messages are especially important in health care because it is so essential that your patients take away the correct meaning of your words—whether the topic is how to take their medications correctly or the importance of following their new diet, or anything else you tell them. In fact, specific body language techniques, which we cover in this chapter, have been found to increase patients' understanding of what their clinicians tell them.

You may not realize the sizable role your body language plays in your interactions with patients. If your body language is seriously misconstrued by patients, it can cause them to switch to another clinician or avoid coming back for follow-up appointments.

Over the past two decades, I have noticed, during coaching sessions with physicians and other clinicians, that many of their behaviors are quite normal and reasonable, given their personality and social style. But a patient who has a different style can easily misinterpret these behaviors. No two patients react quite the same way to you, of course, because of the variations in our perceptions and reactions. Exhibit 4.1 lists some of the most common examples of this misinterpretation of body language that I've observed over the years. The message the patient takes from the clinician's body language is not what was intended to be conveyed at all.

GENERAL GUIDELINES FOR GESTURES

The following tips and guidelines will help you use gestures to your best advantage and avoid the ones that can send a negative message.

Exhibit 4.1. Clinicians' Body Language and Patients' Translations

Clinician Body Language	Patient Translation
Examining x-rays as the patient divulges deep-seated fears	"I'm ignoring your emotional nonsense. Hmmm, what can we fix here?"
Responding to the patient's description of pain with an occasional "OK" or "Um-hmm" without looking up from the chart	"I can't get personally involved. This is purely clinical. You are parts and pieces to me."
Arms folded together over the chest or on the desk while talking with the patient	"Don't even think about getting any closer to my personal space."
Holding the chart against the front of the chest, arms folded over it, while talking with the patient during hospital rounds	"This is top secret information you can't see. You wouldn't understand it anyway; it requires superior intelligence."
Rapid and frequent head nodding while the patient is talking	"OK. OK. Let's get through this! I haven't got all day."
Tapping anything rapidly on the desk: pencil, pen, corner of a prescription pad or envelope	"D'you see how you irritate me? You're taking up my valuable time when I'm in a hurry!"
Listening with no facial expression, no movement of the head or eyes	"You really think I CARE? I'm just enduring this."
Leaning back comfortably in the chair, resting on the lower spine	"Sheesh! You bore me. Maybe I can sleep through this."
Silently and diligently entering data into the computer with back toward the patient	"Oh, are you still here? I thought I was finally alone with all this engrossing stuff."

(continued)

Exhibit 4.1. (continued)

Clinician Body Language	Patient Translation
Looking at the patient through the bottom of bifocal eyeglasses	"Of course I'm looking down my nose at you. I'm vastly more intelligent and powerful than you."
Looking over the top rim of eyeglasses when asking the patient a question	"You'd better have the right answer. Are you thoroughly intimidated yet?"

Body Language Should Convey Openness and Offer Comfort

Nothing should block off the front of your chest area as you face the patient. When arms or hands are held in front of the upper body, we call it a "closed gesture" because you close yourself off from those who are facing you. It's a defensive posture, with the arms fending off unwanted impact from the person in front of you.

Here is an experiment to illustrate the point: sit at the corner of a desk or table with a friend. Sit back, fold your arms solidly over your chest, and say, "Whatever concerns or difficulties you have with this, I'm here to listen and try to help." Use a monotone and no facial expression as you say these words. Next, change your body language. Unfold your arms and rest them on the desk in an open, asymmetrical position. As you face your friend, lean slightly forward and say the sentence again, adding facial and vocal expressions. Ask your friend for feedback as to which version seemed more sincere and reassuring.

Keeping the chest area open, unblocked by folded arms or hands, is generally a friendly, welcoming position. It tends to send the nonverbal message that you are available to help the patient and open to hearing any concerns. You are more likely to appear genuinely interested and caring in this position. It seems to imply, "My heart is open to you." It's a silent but strong message.

Communicating with Today's Patient

Folding your hands together, resting them on the desk in front of you or in your lap, is a variation of the closed gesture. I see this frequently used by clinicians during workshop role plays. The closed circle formed in front of your body as you sit in this position tends to define a sort of boundary of your personal space, setting you apart and closing off the patient. It's as if you're subtly implying, "See this fence around my property? Stay on your side of it."

Again, it's preferable to keep your upper torso open to view, with nothing closing it off—no charts, no folded hands or arms. In this way, you seem approachable and professionally accessible to the patient. Another problem with folded hands is that the thumbs may begin to circle around each other—a classic sign of nervous irritation or of boredom with the person you are listening to.

Just as with arms or hands folded in front, anything else held in front of the chest, such as x-rays, lab results, or a patient chart, also acts as a barrier to open communication. In addition to seeming protective of secret documents, this body position implies a warning that no emotional stuff is tolerated; it's as if the clinician's heart is barricaded by data.

If you look at paintings or statues of the great religious leaders throughout history, they are invariably depicted with their upper torso open to their followers. Whether it is Christ, Buddha, or any other key religious figure, this body position has the effect of encouraging followers to come to them, to be received, enveloped in the caring and comfort that their religion and its leader offer.

Although you are not in a religious setting, as a health care professional you certainly do want to offer comfort to your patients; you do have loyal followers, and you offer a kind of shelter from some of life's deepest concerns. Be aware that your body can convey some of these important images or messages that patients seek, perhaps even at a subliminal level.

Don't "Steeple"

Another form of the closed gesture is called "steepling." The elbows usually rest on the desk, hands held up, with the tips of the fingers touching, as if the hand is forming a steeple tower. The chin may rest in the connected thumbs. Although this is a popular thinking or pondering position, it can also close off the patient from the clinician since the arms and hands form a barrier not only across the upper body but sometimes across the face as well. There is also something forbidding about the "spikes" formed by the pressed-together fingers aimed at the other person.

A Little Off-Center Conveys Comfort

Another strike against these closed gestures is that they are invariably symmetrical. Mehrabian (1972) found that a symmetrical body position was perceived as formal, stiff, and unfriendly. An asymmetrical position appears relaxed, comfortable, and amiable—one arm on the desk and the other on your knee, for example.

Keep Gestures Chest High

To have meaning and significance, gestures should occur in the area of your upper torso—above the waist, below the head. Use gestures to emphasize the important parts of your message.

Keep Elbows Away from Your Sides

If the upper arms and elbows are held close to the body, the resulting gestures involve mostly the lower arm and wrist. Such gestures tend to look weak— passive and powerless. People who appear *authoritative and self-assured* usually use larger gestures and generally take up more physical space than others. You may notice they spread their arms out on a desk or table, or otherwise position their bodies to use more space. A strong, authoritative gesture requires at least some movement of the upper arm as well, to show conviction.

There are times, certainly, when gesturing with the wrist alone is fine and entirely appropriate. But if the tight-to-the-body elbow and the resulting twists of the wrist are the main gestures in one's repertoire, the impression can definitely be one of weakness, ineptness, and passivity. There is a caveat, however. Several years ago, I was conducting a class in presentation skills for the American College of Physician Executives, and a physician took my words about keeping elbows away from the body to the extreme. He delivered his entire speech to the class with his hands on his hips, elbows akimbo! This is a "critical parent" posture and is going much too far in the opposite direction.

Don't Be Overly Expressive

Too many rapid, repeating arm gestures make you look hurried and harried. Use slow, smooth gestures to underline your important points. Gestures that are too big, with too much of the arms moving, can give you the appearance of being unstable or too theatrical. Gestures should be used judiciously, as needed for the effect you want, which is to emphasize the essential points of what you're saying.

Use Gestures That Fortify the Message

All gestures should track with the message. If you say, "It's very important to take all the pills in the bottle," and just give a few vague wafts of your hand, the meaning is lost. But if you use a definite, firm gesture with your hands, such as holding up or firmly tapping the bottle of pills or the prescription, you can underline the importance of taking "*all* the pills." Be sure your gestures are definite, not tentative. They start and finish rather than just fade away.

Pointing Do's and Don'ts

Be careful of pointing—especially at the patient. Instead of a point, use the whole hand, with open fingers that are slightly bent and relaxed. It's a friendly gesture yet still strong. Occasionally you need to point, as in explaining a diagram or x-ray, for example. But generally speaking, avoid pointing at the patient or the patient's family, and try using the open hand gesture instead.

One other tip about pointing: when you are indicating to a patient where to go to find a bathroom or the scales or the front desk, for example, it is rude to extend your pointing hand in front of the patient's face so that the person is looking straight into your arm, wrist, or hand.

Watch Your Hand Signals

Don't rub your face or the front of your chin with your curled fingertips. This may simply be your "I'm thinking about all this, considering it carefully" mannerism. But these positions can also indicate that you don't understand, or that you have doubts about what the person is telling you, or that you flat out don't believe what you are hearing. Watch for these behaviors in patients too, since they can indicate the same concerns on their part.

Avoid covering your mouth with your hand or fingers as you listen to the patient. This can also imply that you don't believe and don't trust the person you are talking with.

Avoid touching or rubbing your nose or your eye area while either you or the patient is talking. Both of these gestures can indicate duplicity, silently suggesting that you are trying to cover up something.

Cupping Your Chin in Your Hands

Supporting your chin with your hands, however, can appear pleasing to patients and can indicate both your interest in them and that you are relaxed and comfortable talking with them. You can undo the value of this position, though, by putting your fingers over your mouth (Larsen and Smith, 1981).

SITTING POSITIONS

Although facial expressions and gestures are commonly thought of as the major components of body language, your sitting position as you talk with your patients is also an essential piece of body language. How you sit can send some of the most important nonverbal messages and can even affect how well your patient listens to you.

Ways to Sit That Say, "I'm Listening"

The clinician leans back in the chair as the patient begins to talk. It's already midafternoon of an unusually busy day. The words of a learned professor back in medical school echo in the back of his mind: "Just sit back

80

in a relaxed position as you talk with the patient, and the patient will then feel relaxed too." So the clinician sits back comfortably, resting on the lower spine, legs crossed. Ahhhh.

Leaning back in a relaxed position, however, tends to be the posture of the more dominant person in an interaction—the one who has more power than the other. Therefore, it is not an appropriate position to indicate your interest and encouragement of partnership with the patient.

Another problem with sitting back is that—although some patients may indeed find it relaxes them too—many more are likely to see this position as too casual, or slouched and disinterested. Patients want to know that you take their health problem seriously. They also want assurance that you bring your fullest effort and energy into all interactions with them.

The best sitting position is to lean slightly forward, with your upper body facing toward the patient. This sitting position was shown to be a significant factor in patient satisfaction by researchers Larsen and Smith (1981), who also determined that when the clinician leaned back, patient satisfaction was lower. Perhaps more important, they found that when physicians used this body position, their patients understood better what they were told. These authors state, "This too seems to support the hypothesis that if the physician directly orients himself toward the patient the patient senses greater interest, listens more intently and retains more information" (Larsen and Smith, 1981, p. 487). We use the term *facing toward* the patient because you don't necessarily have to face the patient directly. Facing them directly is fine with many patients, female patients in particular, but it can be intimidating for others. In addition, men often prefer not to face each other directly when they talk and tend to be more comfortable if they are angled toward each other, together forming a *V* or chevron while talking.

How far you lean in and how much you look the patient in the eye needs to be adjusted according to the patient's preference for a focus on relationship or a focus on task, as we discussed in Chapter Three. Your spine and upper torso don't need to be ramrod straight, but certainly you should look attentive and ready to address the patient's problem. In this position, you are much more likely to appear interested and capable to the patient, conveying what Mehrabian (1972) called "immediacy."

We also suggest you sit on the front two-thirds of the chair seat to instantly achieve this position of immediacy. When you sit on the front two-thirds of the chair, you're likely to lean forward slightly and less likely to slouch. You will probably feel more alert and energetic too.

Be sure you don't have your hands gripping the sides of the chair seat. Adding this little piece of bracing body language can send the message, "I'm waiting for the first opportunity to bolt out of here."

We're not suggesting that you remain in the forward-leaning position all the time, of course. You can certainly sit back and relax from time to time during a patient interview. But consider this as a sort of baseline optimal position for patient interviews. We particularly recommend this sitting position at the beginning and end of the interaction. It is also useful whenever the patient divulges a potentially serious physical or emotional concern. In this case, lean in very slowly and only slightly. If you suddenly bolt forward, the patient may become alarmed, thinking, "Uh-oh. The doctor is *really* worried. Something must be seriously wrong with me."

The Best Position for Arms and Hands

The ideal hand-and-arm position, if you are seated at a table or desk while listening to the patient, is to sit with one arm resting on the desk, the other hand in a relaxed, somewhat open-palm position, also resting on the desk or on your knee. One hand is then ready to write in the chart as needed. Both arms are free to be used, together or singly, for any gestures. You are also in an asymmetrical position, which is more relaxed yet still professional.

Shoulders Signal Your Interest in the Patient

Although eye contact gets a lot of good press in the literature on patient communication, even more important, we believe, is shoulder orientation. Shoulders signal where your main focus is. With your shoulders facing toward the patient, you indicate your interest in listening to the

Communicating with Today's Patient

patient. If your shoulders are facing the chart, however, you indicate that that is your main interest.

You can test the effectiveness of this with a friend or colleague. Sit side by side, both of you facing forward. Turn only your head sideways toward your friend, the rest of your body still facing forward. As you talk, look her in the eye. Next, reposition yourself so that your shoulders and upper torso as well as your head are facing toward your friend. Begin talking again. Now stop and ask for feedback as to which position conveys more of your interest and attention. You will probably find the difference in perception quite remarkable. Shoulder orientation is a powerful piece of body language and has many uses.

Don't Look Sideways at the Patient

Avoid sitting so that your shoulders and upper torso are directly facing the chart, with the patient to your side. This position requires you to glance sideways at the patient when you ask a question. When your shoulders are oriented toward the chart in this way, your silent message is that the chart is your primary interest and the patient is secondary—that it's the data and the medical task you really care about, and the patient is only a means to that end.

Don't Sit Directly Across the Desk from the Patient

Sitting directly across the desk from the patient clearly sets you up as the absolute authority. This position (the parent-child, teacher-student configuration) tells patients that they are to be reverent, passive, and obedient. This is not today's approach to communicating with patients and does not encourage a sense of partnership, comfort, or responsibility in the patient.

How Close to Sit to Patients

Two to four feet is the range that most North Americans like to have between themselves and the person they are interacting with. The optimal distance to be seated from the patient is about three feet, but this distance can vary according to personality, as we discussed in the previous chapter, and can also vary according to the nationality of patients. People who come from families with Northern European or Asian traditions tend to be somewhat formal, with a preference for more social distance and less touching, whereas those from what are called "high touch cultures"— Mediterranean countries or those in Central and South America, for example—tend to be comfortable with closer sitting and standing positions and with more touching in their interactions.

FACIAL EXPRESSIONS

Facial expressions should be appropriate and track with what you are saying or hearing. They are the mark of someone who is responsive, interested, and empathic. Using all the potential in your face for relating to your patient doesn't take any more time and can greatly increase both the quality and the quantity of time, in many patients' perceptions.

Smile at Every Appropriate Opportunity

Seize opportunities to smile whenever it seems appropriate. Smile—or at least have a positive, interested, upbeat expression on your face:

- When you greet the patient at the beginning of the interaction; smile as you say the patient's name
- If you are saying something positive or telling the patient good news
- If the patient or the patient's family reports good news to you
- As you say goodbye to the patient, if this has been a fairly routine visit; smile also at other members of the family as they leave

We're not suggesting a big, toothy, Cheshire Cat grin, just something sized to the occasion. A pleasant smile can have a warming and positive effect on everyone (including you). Keep in mind, however, that patients who are seriously ill often prefer a more serious demeanor.

Avoid Frowning

Some clinicians have the facial habit of frowning while they are working through something puzzling or when they are concentrating intensely. To

84

the patient, this frowning can look as if the clinician is angry with them or disapproving. Many clinicians in our workshop never realized they had this habit until they saw a video replay of themselves.

Take Your Face Out of Park

The clinician is listening intently to what the patient is saying. Silent. Unmoving. So focused on what the patient is saying that concentration is not broken for even a moment to react to the patient as she talks. An immobile face is often referred to as a deadpan expression. That's *deadpan* as in *dead*—showing no sign of life. It can send the message of being austere, stoic, cold. The patient, especially an amiable or expressive one, may secretly want to knock on the clinician's stolid forehead and ask, "Is anyone in there? A real person?" One of our colleagues, Terry Paulson, calls it "putting your face in park."

As you talk with the patient, be sure you respond with a few appropriate facial expressions from the area around the eyes, the forehead, or the mouth. Patients tend to see you as being caring and interested in them as individuals. If you are a highly analytical person, it might be beneficial to ask a more outgoing colleague or friend whether you regularly show some facial response as you are listening to him or her. Many predominantly Analytical people are not aware that they have a low-affect listening style.

EYE CONTACT

An important way of sending nonverbal messages, eye contact also has some essential do's and don'ts attached to its use.

Stay on the Same Eye Level

Whenever possible, remain on the same eye level as the patient. If the patient is on an exam table or a gurney, you can stay at or close to eye level if you perch on a high stool. If the patient is seated or in a hospital bed, it's best if you sit down too. It's preferable to pull up a chair next to the hospital bed, rather than sitting on the patient's bed. Sitting on the bed, though, might be a better alternative than standing. If the sides are up on the hospital bed, let them down as you sit and talk with the patient. Be sure you put the sides back up when you leave.

Whether it is appropriate to sit at the end of the patient's bed depends on the gender, age, and condition of the patient and the caregiver as well. But as a general rule, talking together on the same level is a friendly, caring position that encourages the patient to talk openly with you. It engenders trust, comfort, and partnership. There's an added benefit: patients often perceive the time spent with you as longer—sometimes double the time— if you sit down while you talk with them.

Look from the Center, Not the Corner, of Your Eye

As you look at the patient, try to keep your head facing the patient directly so that your eyeballs are centered in the sockets. Looking out of the corner of your eye is particularly dangerous since it sends a subliminal message that you may not be trustworthy. This is one of the secrets for success that media consultants give their politician clients. If the politician has to look over at someone to the side, the entire head is turned to look at the person rather than keeping the head stationary and just looking out of the corner of the eyes.

A camera close-up of a politician looking out of the corner of the eyes is the kiss of death. Because of the physical proximity and the intimacy of the medical interview, when you talk to a patient, it's a close-up—even without a TV camera. If you are facing the chart, for example, and intermittently look at the patient out of the corner of your eye, this can give you an untrustworthy, shifty-eyed look.

Occasionally we see clinicians sitting with the upper body toward the patient but the head turned ever so slightly away from the patient, eyes slightly angled as they look at the person. Female patients may be especially sensitive to this obliqueness and read it as subtle avoidance. However, male patients, as we mentioned earlier, are often more comfortable with a somewhat angled body and head position for interactions, rather than facing each other straight on.

In the same vein, if you are facing toward your patient and a family member speaks up from the side, try to turn your head toward that person

Communicating with Today's Patient

rather than keeping your head focused on the patient and looking at the family member out of the corner of your eye, which may imply you don't quite trust him or her.

Darting, angled glances can also send the message that you are hurried and agitated. Keep your eyeball centered as much as possible while you look at the patient or family members.

Be Prepared to Shift Focus Back to the Patient

If you are charting and the patient tells you something that is clearly troubling him, be sure you stop. Put down the pen and look at him. This is not the time to write in the chart, or even to read it while perhaps muttering an occasional, absentminded "Um-hmm" to the patient's description of pains and problems.

If your primary focus seems to be on the chart, the patient can feel that you are not really interested in him or that you are insensitive to his psychosocial concerns. Whatever you're facing and looking at is what you're most interested in; at least, that's the perception of many patients we've surveyed informally. If your eyes are focused on the chart as you ask the patient a question or listen to an answer, you're primarily interested in the chart and medical data. Look at the patient when you ask questions or while you listen to the patient's most troubling concerns.

What to Do with Your Glasses

If you wear glasses, avoid looking over the rims or through the bottom of bifocals. Such body language has overtones of a frightening inquisition. It connotes a distinctly authoritarian style, implying a significant difference in status between the clinician and the patient. Rather than encouraging participatory and responsible patients, body language of this sort may encourage the opposite: subservience and dependence. Other patients may find it superior and patronizing and feel resentful.

If a patient divulges something that is obviously profoundly emotional, consider slowly removing your glasses as you listen. This conveys a warm and caring response from you. It tells the patient you can empathize with her and that you are willing to give her personal, individual attention on both the physical and the psychosocial levels. The simple act of taking off and setting aside your glasses is symbolic of leaving your "thinking-examining mode" in order to be available to the patient at a more humanistic, eye-to-eye level.

Subtlety is essential in using many of these techniques. They require a little practice and finesse, perhaps even some feedback and coaching, particularly if these ways of reacting are not naturally part of your communication style.

HEAD MOVEMENTS

Head movements take no extra time and can convey a variety of messages— some positive, and some decidedly negative. Here are some pointers.

Nodding

In just the last few years, my fellow workshop leaders and I have noticed an increase in rapid head nodding during reenactments of patient encounters in our workshops. My guess is that this is a habit recently acquired by busy, time-conscious clinicians who are in a fast-forward mode so much of the time.

It is certainly effective to nod your head occasionally as the patient talks; a sizable body of research backs that up. In fact, we recommend head movement as a key part of active listening (in Chapter Five). But it's better to nod the head somewhat slowly and thoughtfully, and only at key points in the patient's explanation or in yours.

Some clinicians seem to use frequent and rapid head nodding as a form of interruption, as if to signal the patient to stop talking, that they have heard enough of the symptoms, have already made the diagnosis and are now ready to move on to an explanation of the treatment plan. If the patient doesn't pick up the clue and continues to talk about her symptoms, the clinician's head nodding often becomes even more rapid and vigorous, as if to signal nonverbally "I know, I know! I've got the diagnosis. You don't need to go on anymore about symptoms."

Communicating with Today's Patient

This could be a dangerous situation since the majority of clinician errors cited in a recent study were blamed on feeling time pressures or on not considering carefully the patient's stated symptoms (Ely and others, 1995).

Another variation of inappropriate head nodding that we observe frequently is done mostly by very friendly types of clinicians. They nod evenly and not so furtively—but they nod. Continuously! It's almost perpetual motion—nodding as the patient speaks, and it even continues throughout their own explanations as well.

This may be a kind of "Let's be in agreement, okay?" gesture, but it can be very irritating and monotonous to some people. It's as if the head is neurologically stuck in the nodding mode, rather like the little plastic animals stuck onto dashboards or on rear window ledges, perpetually and amiably nodding their heads with every movement of the car. Too much head nodding can give the impression that the clinician is asking not only for agreement but also for approval and acceptance as well. It can have the negative effect of undermining authority, especially with patients who have a predominantly Driving social style. Patients who have an Amiable style, however, may tolerate it well. Some may even *like* it and nod back in the same rhythm.

Again, we definitely recommend some head nodding as you listen to your patient, but nod the head *selectively*, at key points in the patient's explanation or in your own.

Keep Your Chin Level

Try to keep your chin level as you look at the patient. If your chin tends to be raised even slightly, you'll be looking down at the patient, which research shows is clearly a factor in patient dissatisfaction (Larsen and Smith, 1981). If your chin is slightly lowered, with your eyes looking up at the patient, this can give you the appearance of insecurity, shyness, or nervousness. These are acquired mannerisms that clinicians are usually unaware of until they see themselves on videotape.

Don't Put Down a Colleague or Staff Member with Body Language

We often hear of scenarios such as this one. Barbara Barnes has been Dr. Lee's patient for several years. She is a pleasant, middle-aged woman in basically good health, taking only estrogens and thyroid supplements. While Dr. Lee is out of town at a medical meeting, her colleague, Dr. Kasper, is seeing her patients. Ms. Barnes is in today for her regular checkup.

As Dr. Kasper intently reads her chart, he suddenly sighs, purses his lips, and shakes his head side-to-side, clearly exasperated. Ms. Barnes is electrified. The doctor quickly closes the chart, pushes it away to the side of the desk with finality, and announces with a frown, "One thing's clear. We have to change your medications!" How does Ms. Barnes feel? Devastated! She really liked Dr. Lee, and now she fears she's had bad advice and poor-quality care all along.

Dr. Lee returns from her meeting a few days later and finds an urgent request on her desk. It's from Ms. Barnes. She wants her medical files transferred to another health care group across town.

"What happened?" Dr. Lee asks her colleague.

"I only told her we needed to change her medication," Dr. Kasper responds defensively. "Based on her latest blood test, it was time to lower her dose of thyroid meds."

"Did you say anything else to her?" the anxious physician asks. "Anything that might cause her to switch?"

"Look, I just told her about her medication adjustment based on the latest blood tests," he responds, now even more defensive.

Clearly, Dr. Kasper told Ms. Barnes plenty. Through his body language, Dr. Kasper conveyed lack of respect for his physician-colleague and lost her a patient. But when asked about it, he could safely say that he had not *said* anything that was a put-down of Dr. Lee. True, he didn't say it verbally; he said it nonverbally—loud and clear!

If you put down a colleague—even with silent messages conveyed through nonverbal means—you are also demeaning your entire organization. In addition, you can damage your own professional image, since the patient may have a strong emotional attachment to her caregiver and may decide you are the one who is wrong. Or, since you are part of the same organization, any judgment about poor care can extend to you and your entire group or organization as well.

SOME FINAL TIPS

Here are a few tips on how you can incorporate positive body language into your daily visits with patients.

Once a Day, Survey Your Body Language

Toward the end of the day in particular, it can be valuable to take a quick inventory of your body position and facial expressions. This is a time when most of us are not as fresh as we were in the morning. A quick check to see that your nonverbal messages are not sagging a bit in the midafternoon of a busy day can be helpful. Body language can give the impression that you don't care, despite the fact that you do and may only be a bit tired.

Look for Role Models

Observe others who are expressive to see how these techniques are used naturally yet professionally. Try watching the major evening news anchors, many of whom are expressive yet professional and believable. They also need to be likable; they only keep their jobs if their ratings—their satisfaction surveys—are high. They don't use gestures, so they must communicate merely through head movements and facial expressions: a slight raise of the eyebrows, a small squint of the eyes, a head nod, all important body language tools used by these communicators to highlight their important messages.

You can also use many of their same techniques during your explanations to a patient or as a reaction to what a patient is telling you.

Stay Authentic

Do any of these techniques feel a little like show biz? Like acting a part? Then don't use them. At least not right away. Never use any facial expressions or

Exhibit 4.2. Positive Body Language and Translations

Clinician Body Language	Patient Translation
Sitting up, comfortably, with a slight forward lean of your upper torso toward the patient	"I'm bringing my full energy, interest, and attention to our meeting as well as my best efforts."
Maintaining appropriate eye contact, being particularly careful to look at the patient if he or she divulges something that is emotionally troubling	"You and I have an important and positive professional connection. We'll work together. You can bring me your concerns, both physical and emotional."
Shoulders and upper torso facing or angled toward the patient	"You are the primary focus, not the chart, not the computer. They are of secondary importance, and I will turn to them as needed. You have my fullest attention. I respect and value you as a unique individual."
Nodding the head selectively and at key points as the patient talks	"I'm listening, and I'm interested in what you are saying."
A smile as appropriate	"I'm really happy to see you, and I look forward to working with you."
Occasional facial expression that shows your (appropriate) reaction to what the patient is telling you	"You and I are a team, and I respect what you have to tell me. I hope that you feel comfortable telling me anything that concerns you."
Upper torso not closed off by arms or charts or medical equipment whenever possible	"I am available to give you my fullest professional attention. I am always approachable."

gestures or body positions that feel phony to you. There's a high probability they also seem phony to the patient.

What you can do, however, is begin at once to practice these skills in a safe, relaxed environment first. For example, you might try using a few more facial expressions and gestures than usual as you talk with family, friends, or colleagues. Gradually, the techniques may become part of your natural style, integrated into your personality, not put on just for the sake of making a good impression. You can make significant adjustments in your style with some effort, awareness, and practice.

Get Some Feedback

Now that you've read this chapter on nonverbal communication, we suggest you casually ask a friend or colleague to read over Exhibit 4.2, which lists some proven nonverbal techniques that deliver positive signals to patients' "perception radar." Then ask for some candid comments as to which nonverbal skills you need to work on. Better yet, seek the help of a professional coach for physicians and other health care professionals. This kind of honest feedback can be valuable in the long run.

POSITIVE BODY LANGUAGE

The body-language communication techniques listed in Exhibit 4.2 send the message to your patients that you care about them and are on track with them. If you're using these techniques already, consider this a 3,000-mile checkup.

These communication tips can ensure that your words and actions send a consistent message. Before most of us feel motivated to work on improving a skill, we first have to be aware that we need to do so. Awareness often comes through a significant, painful event: a complaint, a poor review, even a lawsuit. We hope you can use the pointers and suggestions in this chapter and throughout the rest of the book as preventive measures to make sure that such painful events never occur.

By using positive nonverbal communication techniques, you can demonstrate your capacity to understand and identify with the feelings of your patients, thereby improving or reinforcing your relationships with them.

Now that we have reviewed both verbal and nonverbal communication techniques, let's move on to the equally important topic of listening techniques that help you quickly gather accurate information from your patients.

Communicating with Today's Patient

CHAPTER 5

Listening Techniques for Faster, More Accurate Diagnoses

Your talent for careful, insightful listening is more essential than ever today. In a time of cost containment and utilization reviews, the array of diagnostic tests is no longer the ready option of years past. Your ability to listen to the patient to determine what is really occurring is a critical factor in making an accurate diagnosis.

In three out of four cases, your final diagnosis is derived from what the patient tells you during the history-gathering process and then is backed up by the physical exam and lab tests. The physical exam alone leads to the diagnosis in only about 12 percent of patients, and the laboratory investigations produce the diagnosis in only 11 percent of patients (Peterson and others, 1992). Other researchers rank the history much higher as the major source for a diagnosis, as much as 82–90 percent in some studies (Gruppen, Wooliscroft, and Wolf, 1988).

Therefore, your skill as a diagnostician is determined in large part by the acuity of your listening skills. Physician-philosopher Sir William Osler underscored the importance of listening when he advised physicians to listen to their patients because they would tell the physician the diagnosis (Osler, 1899).

In this chapter, we cover listening techniques, some of which may be new and others that can be added to what you're already using. All help you glean essential information from your patients in an efficient manner. These techniques have another advantage in that they also strengthen your connection with the patient at the same time.

THREE KEY LISTENING SKILLS

The first three techniques are active, reflective, and empathic listening. Each has a specific look and sound to it; each has a specific goal and a particular outcome.

The goal of active listening is to respond to what the patient is telling you, through your actions such as facial expression and brief vocal utterances, which clearly indicate that you are attentive to what the patient is saying about the physical and emotional concerns.

The goal of reflective listening is to let your patient know you are listening, by reflecting back what the patient told you. It encourages the patient to clarify further or expand on the information and allows you to check that you accurately understood what the patient told you.

The goal of empathic listening is to indicate clearly that you are interested in the psychosocial aspects of the patient's illness along with the physical; this also tends to strengthen the relationship. We describe how you can use these techniques at the most advantageous points in the interaction for greatest effectiveness.

ACTIVE LISTENING

Active listening involves brief responses, body movements, and facial expressions that are typically associated with listening interactively, such as a smile or a nod of the head in reaction to what the patient says. It also means using vocal responses (a murmured "Um-hmm" or "I see"), which give the patient auditory proof that you are listening. Through these brief actions—both body language and vocal responses—patients can see and

Communicating with Today's Patient

hear that you are listening, that you follow and understand their descriptions of the illness. Active listening is also a good way to express your empathy with their situation; even something as simple as a slight movement of your eyes or eyebrows can be effective, properly used.

If you have a naturally responsive personality, chances are you already use these active listening techniques instinctively. If you are somewhat less responsive, you might try to incorporate some of these behaviors. You will probably have to work at it since they may not come naturally. Clinicians who are generally focused more on the task to be done than on the relationship often tend to listen with less affect and a rather cool, formal style of interacting. You may feel comfortable adopting only a few of these behaviors, but that can still make a difference and be a significant improvement.

Here are several ways you can make sure that your patients see and hear you listening.

Facial Expression That Says, "I'm Listening"

Use facial expressions to react to what patients tell you—facial expressions that typically signal "I'm attentive to what you say; and furthermore, I'm interested." You might include a slight widening of the eyes or a lift of the eyebrows to show interest, or a frown or slight wincing motion of the eyes if the patient describes a painful situation. Nothing dramatic is needed, just subtle reactions, used sparingly, to what the patient is describing, such as nodding occasionally, at key points as the patient talks.

Check Your Body Language

Lean slightly forward toward your patients as you listen. As we mentioned in Chapter Four on body language, this conveys that you are bringing your energy and attention to the conversation.

Keep your shoulders oriented toward the patient. Again, female patients are generally comfortable with shoulders facing directly toward them, whereas male patients may prefer a slightly angled position but still with shoulders toward them.

Give Vocal Confirmation

Another way to use active listening is through brief, murmured acknowledgments ("Um-hmm," "I see," "Yes"). Patients "hear" that you are listening to them and understanding their meaning. These murmured acknowledgments also connote that "we're on the same track." They facilitate and encourage your patients to tell you important information.

These utterances, however, can have the opposite effect if not used correctly. As a surgeon in a recent workshop commented, "This is exactly how I sound—'Um-hmm . . . Yeah . . . Sure . . .'—when I want to read the newspaper and my wife just keeps yammering on and on about something. Makes her furious." It's true. These murmurs *can* have a negative effect if not used correctly.

What makes the difference? Body language and vocal tone give away the attitude of the listener. If you have no eye contact, or if you're doing something else—reading a chart, adjusting an instrument, or organizing your desktop—as you utter these um-hmms, it implies to the patient, "I'm only pretending to listen to you. I really wish you'd be quiet and let me do what I'm doing, which is far more interesting than your boring prattle." Patients (just like spouses) get the clear perception you're not listening, but merely responding mechanically to hold them at bay. The verbal message has to track with the body language to be believed.

Coupled with matching body language, however, these active listening utterances ("Um-hmm," "Oh," "I see," or just an understanding "Yes") can signal to your patients that you are focused on them; the verbal and nonverbal messages are all in sync. Patients see and hear you listening with their senses and tend to remember it.

Make Eye Contact

Look at patients particularly when they tell you something they believe is important information about their illness. Whether or not you think it is important, look at them as you listen respectfully to their viewpoint.

Listening to Patients on the Telephone

Your voice is your only representative on the telephone. Since no body language is involved, your voice conveys the total impact of what you say and of how you relate to the patient. Active listening acknowledgments are especially important on the telephone. If you are silent as you listen, the patient may quickly surmise that you're not paying attention, or not interested, or even doing something else—like opening mail or checking stock quotations on the Web. Or the patient might assume that your silence reflects your disapproval or disbelief of what you are hearing. Let patients know—through the brief acknowledgments of active listening, such as "I see," "sure," "yes," "OK," and so forth—that you are still "connected" over the telephone lines—connected personally as well as electronically.

Using active listening is especially important for those clinicians who have a task-focused approach and prefer information gathering over relationship building. People with the Analytical social style tend to listen silently with few, if any, interjections, which they may perceive as being interruptions and thus undesirable. They're not. Those interjections are part of listening interactively and are quite comfortable to those patients who put an emphasis on relationships.

REFLECTIVE LISTENING

Reflective listening is when you respond to patients by repeating or reflecting back key parts of what they've just told you. It's also an auditory confirmation to patients that you are listening and attentive, but is longer than the simple "uh-huh" of active listening. In addition, reflective listening conveys to patients that their role in this history-gathering process is important and valued.

A Quick Way to Check for Accuracy of Understanding

Reflective listening is a good way to confirm that you've correctly understood the patient's description of symptoms and main concerns by repeating back important parts of what that patient said. Occasionally, reflective listening serves as an accuracy check for patients as well. As they listen to you repeat back what they said, they can then consider it for a moment and perhaps assess whether or not what they told you is really accurate. Perhaps a bit inflated? Or not as strongly stated as it should have been? Reflective listening allows patients to review their own characterization of the illness. It can be an accuracy check for both of you.

Be Sure They Hear You Listening

Here are two brief examples of reflective listening:

> Patient: Well, the pain usually starts on the left side.
> Clinician: On the left side.

> Patient: I noticed the nausea about an hour after taking that medicine.
> Clinician: About an hour later. I see.

Instead of repeating, you might prefer to paraphrase:

> Patient: I seem to feel the headaches most when I get home at night and there's *so much* to do but I'm just *too exhausted* to do it.
> Clinician: So the headaches are worse when you come home . . . *really tired* . . . and there's *still* work to do.

There are three levels of listening benefit in this example:

- The patient hears you listening.
- You check that you understood what the patient told you.
- The patient senses your empathy and legitimization of the problem when you slightly emphasize the words *exhausted* and *still*.

Rephrase to Check for Clarity

Another way to use reflective listening is to rephrase, often in the form of a question:

"From your point of view, then, . . . ?"

"So, as you see it . . ."

"You mean . . . ?"

"In other words, it sounds as if . . ."

"Let's see if I have this straight. Your main concern about the surgery is . . ."

"This is what I think I hear you saying. . . ."

If you need clarification from the patient, try:

"Help me to be clearer on this. You said . . . "

"You seem to be having . . ."

If you're a little off base, the patient can correct your impression ("Well, actually, it's more like . . .").

Summarize What You Heard

Instead of using questions, you can also put your reflective response in the form of a summary statement: "Sounds as if this has been a continuing problem for you" or "So, it sounds as if this particular medication isn't doing what we hoped it would." This wraps up, succinctly, the essentials of what the patient has been telling you. However, be sure it is not oversimplified or trivialized in any way.

Use Reflective Listening as a Wrap-up

Still another advantage of the summary statement is that it can also serve as a smooth segue when you need to move to the next section of the visit, such as when you are ready to give the patient your suggested treatment plan: "So, from what you tell me, you've really had a lot of discomfort with this sinusitis. It's been an ongoing problem, and I can hear how frustrating it is for you. To help you get some relief from your symptoms, I'm going to recommend . . ." With this last sentence as a transition, you smoothly move on to the treatment recommendation.

Use the Patient's Vocabulary

Use the patient's terminology, as appropriate:

> "You mentioned a tight band around your head. Does that tight band . . . ?"

> "That knife in your chest—when do you feel it most?"

> "What seems to bring on this feeling of an elephant sitting on your chest?"

Use the patient's terminology for discussing gastrointestinal or urological concerns, such as elimination or sexual functions, if that seems appropriate. Your patient may understand, "When you have to pee" better than "When you have to urinate." Using the patient's language can also reduce the level of social distance between the two of you, putting you on an approachable plane. This often helps to reinforce the relationship.

There may be times, of course, when it's just too uncomfortable or unprofessional for you to use the patient's terminology. In this case, you might use the patient's term, followed by, "or, as we say, urinate . . . ," and after that use your preferred term. (For more on this, see the section on medical jargon in Chapter Six.)

Using the patient's language is also contraindicated when dealing with a teenager. Pre- and postadolescents tend to be turned off by adults who try to speak their language. They often see through it, resent it, and lose respect for the adult. Experts on dealing with teenagers tell us that when an adult uses words, phrases, and even pronunciations that are typically used by teens, they react negatively, saying, in effect, "Act your own age. Sound like an adult!" (Tannen, 1986, p. 106).

When Reflective Listening Backfires

Patients who attempt to tell about their main health concerns in the first few minutes of the visit are interrupted by physicians after only eighteen seconds, on average, according to an often-cited study conducted by Howard Beckman, M.D., and Richard Frankel, M.D., of Wayne State University School of

Medicine (Beckman and Frankel, 1984). Many of those interruptions were actually reflective listening responses that were used too soon.

Here's an example of how it works. The patient begins to tell her story:

Patient: Well, I've been having headaches at night and—

Clinician: Is it a sharp or a dull pain?

Patient: Dull, mostly, and—

Clinician: On the left or the right?

Patient: On the right—

and they are off on the track of the headaches, describing, defining, delineating them intently. The problem is that this is not really what brings the patient in today. The headache is just the first thing she mentions—and the first thing the clinician seizes on. The patient then follows the clinician's lead, dutifully answering each question, probably thinking the doctor knows best. But at the end of the visit, that patient often brings up, at last, the real concern, and the two have to start all over, or schedule another visit. This is the classic "oh-by-the-way" dilemma.

That's why we strongly recommend that you avoid reflective listening for the first several minutes—two at least—during the patient's presentation of chief concerns, and use only active listening occasionally, such as facial expressions, nods, or very brief murmurs of acknowledgment. These facilitating responses allow the patient to tell of any other pressing concerns. Keep in mind that the first symptoms the patient mentions may not be first in importance—that is, not what actually brought her in. Avoid any reflective or empathic listening, and use only active listening during those first two minutes when the patient tells you "the story of her illness."

Avoid Conditioning the Patient to Passivity

One caveat about interrupting: any time you interrupt a patient, particularly in midsentence, it is a way of subtly taking on the superior or dominant role. It can condition the patient to be passive, to limit his responsibility for the flow of information, and to wait until you ask a question before responding. Patients are often vaguely resentful if you do this and may see you as domineering and rude.

EMPATHIC LISTENING

Empathic listening addresses the emotional component of the patient's illness or difficulty. Although there is limited, precious time with each patient, we have been able to demonstrate in our workshops, with feedback from those in the patient role, that it takes as little as thirty to sixty seconds to delve into the emotional component of the illness. Researchers found that affective responses from the clinician even shortened the consultation time in some cases (van Dulmen, Verhaak, and Bilo, 1997). The valuable information you receive can bring a complete picture of the emotional underpinnings of the ailment, often a contributing factor.

Empathic responses include:

- "That must have been difficult for you."
- "I'm sorry to hear that."
- "You seem anxious."
- "You seem concerned."
- "You seem uncomfortable."
- "I can understand why that would make you feel nervous (sad, worried, happy)."
- "So that news made you feel sad."

Listening Empathically Is "Doing Something"

A physician in one of the workshops, who worked mostly in a retirement setting, complained that his patients were all so ill and had so many problems when they came in that he couldn't just keep saying these phrases to all the patients he saw during the day. I responded, "Why not?" If all his patients need that empathy, why not give it to them? There are many other routine things he did repeatedly through the course of a day; why not add this important, often therapeutic response and help those senior patients feel better? "But this isn't doing anything for them!" he retorted. Oh yes it is—at a psychosocial level, if not a physical level. Talk and empathy can often be the most valuable intervention—just what the *patient* ordered.

As you are no doubt aware, some of your patients—especially lonely seniors who seldom get out—view a visit to the clinic as one of the important social events of the week or month. They want and often need to take some time to just connect with you through conversation, a little small-talk time. This can be a potent medication, to have someone who listens to them, empathizes, and treats them as important individuals.

Listening as a Bonding Agent

At the point where patients—of any age—are able to open up and share their fears or their sadness, which they may have been keeping inside, this emotional unloading can quickly establish a therapeutic alliance with you. The patient's resulting trust and sense of connection surely continues to enhance your ability to gain information. Such emotional bonding or connecting with the patient carries a significant benefit, in providing quality care for your patient and in your own professional satisfaction as well. In addition, the patient's loyalty often extends to others in your group or organization. On a pragmatic note, many researchers have noted a strong association with lessened risk of malpractice whenever patients feel a positive emotional connection with the clinician.

Lanny points out that if a patient doesn't feel listened to in a caring way, the patient becomes frustrated and may well leave your office and never come back. The relatives and friends of that patient can hear about it, he says, and it can be devastating to a practice.

The Most-Often-Missed Opportunity

Despite all the evidence that listening in a caring way is vitally important in patient communication, this is the most frequently missed opportunity I have observed during fifteen years of presenting Desmond Medical Communications workshops to physicians and other clinicians. The appropriate moment for empathic listening goes unnoticed, and instead a task-oriented response is used. Here are some examples:

Patient: I've just been under so much stress lately.

Clinician: Are you still taking your blood pressure medication?

A preferable response by the clinician would be, "I'm sorry to hear that," "What stress have you been experiencing lately?" or "Tell me more about that."

Another example: a patient says, "I've been having terrible headaches from my allergies for the past two weeks, and nothing seems to relieve it anymore! It's driving me crazy."

In our workshop role plays, my trainers and I hear as the most typical response to statements of pain and suffering such as this, "OK" or "Uh-huh," with no responsive affect in either the clinician's face or the voice.

This type of response is completely off track from what the patient has just described. A week of piercing sinus headache is *not* OK with the patient! Flat, low-affect responses such as "OK" or "I see" can be translated by the patient to mean "data entered" or "detached and uncaring." It would take only a few seconds to respond, "That must be difficult" or "That's a long time to have constant sinus headache pain." If you want to express your empathy but are concerned that it might interrupt or divert the patient's story of the illness, you can respond silently just through subtle facial reactions indicating your empathy.

Another example: when a patient tells you that a family member died, the response "I'm sorry to hear that" is usually appropriate and kind. It is certainly more caring than what we often hear in our workshop role plays: "Oh? What did he die of?" This response smacks of "I need this for my records. The medical task is top priority here." If the information is important for reasons of possible family predisposition, give the empathic response—"I'm sorry to hear that"—*first* and then ask about cause of death.

Of all the listening skills that need to be improved among clinicians generally, this is probably the most prominent. It's easy to improve, and a

Communicating with Today's Patient

major part is simply having heightened awareness of the opportunities as well as the benefits. Don't whiz over the emotional aspects of what the patient is telling you. Don't dismiss those litanies of pain and discomfort from a patient with a perfunctory, "OK." Take two or three seconds to acknowledge that discomfort.

Encouraging Patients

Listen for places where you can interject a bit of encouragement or a pat on the back:

"Looks like you've really made an effort to . . ."

"You've come a long way in . . ."

"I think you're showing a big improvement in the area of . . ."

"It's clear this means a lot to you."

"I certainly support you in . . ."

"It's clear you're really working on this, even though it hasn't been easy."

Encouragement comes from the Latin *cor*, or heart, meaning to give heart. The dictionary defines *encourage* as inspire to continue on a chosen course, which sounds a lot like compliance or adherence. It takes very little time to give a few encouraging words to a patient, but the effect can be long lasting. Your words can echo in the patient's mind at the very moment they are most needed: weeks later, when discouragement and "Oh, why bother with all this?" creeps in.

Dealing with a Weeping Patient

If the patient begins to sob, the simple gesture of passing a tissue to the patient can be remarkably therapeutic and symbolic of your caring. Yet many clinicians pass up this simple opportunity to show their concern for the patient, probably because of preference for a rational, objective approach to patient interaction and discomfort with a strong, emotional response.

Some clinicians prefer to let the patient cry without handing over a tissue. They feel the message to the patient in not intervening in this way is that crying is good, therapeutic, OK to do, and not something embarrassing to be swept away by a tissue.

But many others who have themselves been in the weeping-patient's chair strongly prefer this simple comforting gesture; we do also, particularly when it is carried out gently and quietly.

During a weeping-patient role play in one of our workshops, the clinician quickly and efficiently reached over—the instant the tears began—grabbed a box of tissues, and loudly plopped it in front of the patient. Then the clinician sat back as if saying, "There! Now, get a hold on yourself, for heaven's sake." Technique is everything.

It's also important not to offer a tissue too soon. Wait until tears actually come. If you offer a tissue as the eyes are just beginning to redden or fill up, your gesture could be misinterpreted to indicate that you'd prefer the patient get rid of any tears—immediately—with a tissue.

Men are generally conditioned not to cry, yet we know that crying can be as therapeutic for them as it is for women as a means of releasing their grief or sorrow. If a man does cry, particularly if the clinician is female, it can be very sensitive to say, "You're feeling a very *strong* emotion just now, and that's important." You can add, if it seems appropriate, "So, I can leave you in privacy for a while, if you prefer. I'll be right out in the hall, whenever you're ready for me to come back in." Characterizing crying as "strong" can put it in a positive light for male patients, who may be embarrassed at their show of supposedly feminine emotions.

WELL-MEANING RESPONSES THAT TURN PATIENTS OFF

It's important to acknowledge the patient's discomfort, but it's also important not to add to it inadvertently. Here are some caveats.

Be Careful of Misplaced Sympathy

Be sure that you are fairly certain, from the patient's words and body language, that she is actually experiencing distress before you say, "That must

Communicating with Today's Patient

be difficult." For example, a patient who has a handicapped daughter was describing a recent trip with her. As she described their travels, the clinician responded, "That must have been difficult." The clinician's sympathetic response, based on the assumption that such a child would be a burden, was not received well at all. Instead, the patient was offended, since she finds the child a great joy and delights in taking special care of her. Be sure the emotional component is explicit in the patient's words or implicit in the body language before you respond in this way.

Don't Tell the Patient How to Feel

If the patient moans, "Oh, I'm just so nervous about this surgery next week," many well-meaning clinicians respond, "Oh now, there's no need to worry!"

Or if the patient reveals that "I just feel so sad since my wife died. I don't know what I'm going to do!" the response we often hear is, "Well now, there's no need to feel that way. You have a lot be grateful for." That kind of well-meaning response actually demeans the patient's feelings. It invalidates the feelings and implies that you know better how the patient should feel.

For people who come from families where it was not considered appropriate to show feelings openly, this can be very distressing to hear. A better response, an empathic listening response, is "I can understand that you'd be concerned about surgery. What I can tell you is . . ." or "It must be very difficult losing your wife after so many happy years together. I can certainly understand why you'd feel sad, Mr. _____." This kind of response tells patients you are on frequency with them and you acknowledge what they are going through. It doesn't mean you bear their sorrows and pain yourself, but rather that you acknowledge the difficulties they are facing. This can be very comforting for patients, validating their emotional reaction to their pain.

You Really Don't Know How They Feel

If the patient divulges a strong emotion (such as the one we've just mentioned: "Oh, I'm so nervous about this surgery next week!") and the clinician responds, "Oh, I know just how you feel," this too is inappropriate. Unless the clinician has also faced and experienced the same surgery, there is no possibility of knowing how the patient feels. The reply often leaves patients angry, thinking *Oh no, you don't!*

Another patient might say, "Oh, I'm really worried about what my husband will say about this. He doesn't want us to have any more children, and here I am pregnant again." For a clinician to say, "I understand how you feel" in this case is absurd (especially if the clinician is male). No one except this patient knows how she feels.

A much better response would be "I can understand why you would feel concerned." Note that the key changes are adding the words *can understand* and *why you would*. In the second version, you are agreeing with the legitimacy of her reaction and showing your empathy regarding her concerns. That is a much more believable and patient-pleasing response.

Although they are essential, the three types of listening that we've covered so far—active, reflective, and empathic—are not the only useful listening techniques. In the remainder of this chapter, we review how you can use open- and closed-ended questions to greatest advantage, how to prompt the patient, and how to be alert for emotional clues.

OPEN-ENDED QUESTIONS

If you have ever made a house call, you probably noticed that you learned a lot about the patient and the patient's illness just by going into the home. Chances are you learned far more about what might be contributing factors in the patient's illness than if the patient had come to see you in your office. Few clinicians make house calls today, but there is a way you can vicariously enter the patient's personal world. The closest thing to a house call we have in contemporary health care is the open-ended question. You subtly ask your patient to let you into his or her home—into the psychosocial environment—for a look around, so that you can gain greater understanding of the patient and the possible factors in the illness.

Communicating with Today's Patient

Advantages of Using Open-Ended Questions

Open-ended questions have a number of benefits in a clinical setting. Patients are encouraged to take an active role in the interaction rather than a passive stance. They are often forthcoming, acting in partnership during the history-gathering process.

Another advantage of using open-ended questions, especially at the beginning of the interview, is that this is an adult-to-adult mode of communicating rather than the parent-child style of closed-ended questions.

These questions give you an inside track on the patient's health beliefs about the ailment—critical information for all your future communications. Understanding the patient's beliefs about the illness is particularly valuable as a predictor of how well the patient will adhere to the medications or treatment plan you prescribe.

An open-ended question also signals to patients that they don't need to wait for your questions but can volunteer important information at any point. Studies show that when the patient does the interrupting of the physician, the patient usually brings forth significant information, which may be important in making an accurate diagnosis (Realini, Kalet, and Sparling, 1995).

In addition, patients are more likely to feel a partnership with you if they're part of the team. This has even greater benefits for both of you, especially the patient. The studies of Kaplan, Greenfield, and Ware (1989) indicate that "a more active role in a visit with a physician can relate to a greater sense of control over the disease and therefore a better health outcome."

Bringing in Another Expert

In our workshops, we often watch a video of an interview between an authoritarian clinician and a patient, characterized by mostly hard-driving, dominating, closed-ended questions. Then we view another video of a more affiliative interaction, an interview on a more equal plane. The question then put to the group is, "How many experts do we have in each of these scenes?" Clearly there is one "expert" in the first video example and two in the second. A clinician has expertise about the textbook manifestations of this disease, but the patient is the expert on how the disease shows up in his or her body.

To draw on this patient expertise, the open-ended question is your best ally. Such questions not only invite an answer but also connote respect for and genuine interest in the other person's point of view. If the physician dominates the talk of the visit, either in actual talk or in emotional tone, the patient is likely to be less satisfied (Bertakis, Roter, and Putnam, 1991).

Receive Rather Than Take a History

We encourage the concept of "receiving" a history rather than "taking" a history. It's a different mind-set, but far more appropriate for today's patients and in today's health care environment. It relies on asking questions with the skill and finesse of an investigative reporter coupled with the gentleness of a caring friend. It also means asking well-constructed open-ended questions to get the patient to give information so you can receive it. Many clinicians are concerned about the Pandora's box syndrome, but several researchers indicate that this doesn't seem to take up more time, or very little more—only sixty to ninety seconds. This has also proved to be the case over the years in the timed role plays during Desmond Medical Communications workshops.

Jump-Starting Open-Ended Questions

It's helpful to understand the anatomy of an open-ended question. How do you begin one? You already know that open-ended questions cannot be answered yes or no or with another short answer. But knowing the concept is one thing, and knowing how to switch rapidly from open-ended to closed-ended questions is another—a valuable skill that will come in handy several times a day.

Open-ended questions begin with the words *who, what, when, where, why,* and *how.* Notice these are all adjectives or adverbs: "Who is home to help you?" "What seems to make it worse?" "When do you generally take this medicine?" "Where do you feel the pain most?" "How does exercise affect this?"

Classically, *why* is also included in the list, but it can be perceived as judgmental ("Why did you come to urgent care?" "Why did you stop taking the antibiotic?" "Why did that worry you?"). We suggest avoiding *why* questions, instead rephrasing them with openers such as *what* or *when* to get the same information: "When did you stop taking the antibiotic?" or "What was occurring that caused you to stop the medication?" or "What was your main concern about that?" These are softer and less pointed questions than *why*, which has an aura of authoritarianism about it—a bit of the critical-parent feel.

Questions That Say, "I Want to Hear You"

Start the patient interview with an open-ended question such as, "How can I help you today?" or "What brings you in today?" Open-ended questions foster detailed, broad-spectrum answers rather than single-word responses. It encourages the patient to open up to you. It's also a friendly way to begin instead of a closed-ended get-down-to-business opening such as "I see from your chart you're having arm pain. When did it start?" or "So, Dr. Gage tells me you've had dizziness. Did that start recently?"

The Optimal Time to Use Open-Ended Questions

Use mostly open-ended questions at the beginning of the history to get the patient talking ("When did you first notice the dizziness?" "What do you mean by a queasy stomach?"). This open-ended questioning not only invites patients to open up but also shows that you respect their observations about their health situation and encourage input and active participation. Although valuable at almost any point during your interactions with patients, open-ended questions used early in the history-gathering process seem to bring the best results.

Reliable, All-Purpose Question Starters

An excellent way to start off questions that can be used in a variety of situations is, "How would you describe . . . ?"—for example, "How would you describe the pain?" "How would you describe the relationship between you and your mother?" ". . . the situation at home?" ". . .your experience with . . . ?" This questioning phrase, "How would you describe . . . ?" works effectively in many situations. Said in a soft tone and with slow pacing, it can get you through some difficult situations where you need the information but are not sure whether the patient wants to talk about the topic. An opener such as "How would you describe your relationship with your husband?" (or "your sexual relationship") is much more likely to get a response than just asking, "Is there anything else you'd like to talk about?" It's too easy for the patient to say, "Nope," to that one, especially if the topic is embarrassing to this person.

Another very useful starter for difficult questions is this variation of the one above: "What has been your experience with . . . ?" This can also be useful in situations that might be a bit touchy for the patient.

Here's an actual example of how it can be used effectively. A middle-aged man named Stan, who had just lost fifty pounds after years of trying unsuccessfully to lose weight, went to see his new doctor when he changed HMO plans. The man still weighed more than two hundred pounds, on a medium frame, but he was quite pleased with himself for shedding those fifty pounds. After a perfunctory greeting, the first thing his new doctor said to him was, "Well, I'll tell you one thing straight off. You have *got* to lose some weight!" Stan got up, walked out, and never came back.

Had the physician used the question we suggest here (and if he'd looked more carefully at the chart first), he could have asked, "What's been your experience with weight gain and weight loss over the years?" and Stan might still be his patient.

Our Recommended Version of an Old Favorite

"Do you have any idea what might be causing this?" "What do *you* think might be causing this?"

Many clinicians have been trained to use this type of question. We hear it often in our workshop role plays. In the first version, it is closed-ended and can too easily be answered with a shrug or an "I don't know." The advantage of the second form is that it's open-ended, starting with *what,* and it affirms that the patient's assessment of the situation is important. It also urges patients to share pertinent information—even something they might be more comfortable withholding.

The problem with this popular type of question is that some patients may reply (or think), "Well if I knew, I wouldn't need to come see you, would I? That's what I'm paying for. To have *you* tell me what's causing my problem." Driving or Expressive patients in particular are likely to say that straight out.

We recommend an alternative approach that maintains the benefits of this question but removes the well-don't-you-know? aspect. Add a piece to the front to give the rationale for your question: "Mr. ___, over the years I've found that many of my patients have a very good sense of (*or* some very good ideas as to) what might be causing their problems. So, I'd like to ask you: What do you think might be causing this?" Or "So I'll ask you: What do you think might be involved here [or "contributing to the problem"]?" Vary the specific words to fit your own style, but if you use the introductory sentence first, you have all the benefits of this excellent question and avoid the potential problems.

Although we strongly recommend using open-ended questions, there are times when closed-ended questions are appropriate; we explore this topic in the next section.

CLOSED-ENDED QUESTIONS

Closed-ended questions are specific and focused. They don't encourage a broad-spectrum response but rather are answered with yes, no, or very few words. Closed-ended questions have quite a different character from open questions; they can be useful if skillfully employed. They should be used carefully, however, since they can have a negative impact on patients.

Advantages of Closed-Ended Questions

The closed-ended question can give you quick, narrowly focused information that can be tremendously useful at a critical point later in the history-gathering process, or in a review of systems, for example, or when making a final diagnosis. They are a fast way to zero in on the problem at hand and eliminate other possibilities.

Jump Starts for Closed-Ended Questions

It's important to know how to start them off so you can quickly switch from closed to open questions as needed. Closed-ended questions typically begin with:

Is it . . . ?

Does it . . . ?

Do you . . . ?

Are you . . . ?

Have you . . . ?

Can you . . . ?

All are verbs, usually forms of *to do, to have,* and *to be (able).*

Examples of closed-ended questions are "Do you notice this at particular times of day?" "Have you had regular menstrual cycles?" "Can you walk without pain?" "Are you able to stand up quickly without feeling dizzy?"

Be aware that many closed-ended questions begin with *any.* The true beginning of verb and pronoun ("Have you . . ." "Are you . . ." "Do you . . .") has simply been truncated, and the question begins with *any:* "Any trouble sleeping at night?" "Any difficulty holding down food?" "Any problems with the medication?" (Any chance of framing these as open-ended questions?)

Ideally, you have the beginnings of open-ended and closed-ended questions so clearly in mind that you can easily switch back and forth, using open questions at the right time and closed ones when they are more appropriate.

If possible, during the next few days notice how often you use closed-ended questions. At least one-third to one-half of your questions

Communicating with Today's Patient

probably can be phrased as open-ended, particularly in the initial stages of the history. I have noticed a pronounced tendency in our workshops for the physicians and other clinicians to use closed-ended questions predominantly.

Dangers of Closed-Ended Questions

If closed-ended questions are used too early in the interaction, patients can become passive and less apt to volunteer information about either the physical or the emotional aspects of the disease, both of which are important in your final diagnosis.

A barrage of closed-ended questions can leave the patient feeling frustrated and shut out. Not only does this kind of questioning condition the patient to a passive stance, less likely to open up, but it also makes the clinician appear authoritarian, controlling, and superior, with little interest in having a partnership with the patient. The arrangement is clearly "I ask, you answer." If you must ask closed questions, at least mix in a few open-ended questions to keep the patient involved and to bring out the information you need.

Another danger is that a staccato series of closed-ended questions may give the patient the perception that you are rushing through the appointment (what we call the revolving-door syndrome). The patient can also interpret this to mean you are uncaring and disinterested.

Announce a Series of Closed-Ended Questions

Whenever you do need to use many closed-ended questions in a sequence, announce them first. One way to do this is by saying, "Now I'm going to ask you several questions that can help us focus on some of the additional information we need to have here. Do you . . . ?" or, "Mr. Cusak, I'd like to ask you a series of questions now, which will help me determine more precisely what we're dealing with. Does this pain . . . ?"

When the questions are in a series, as during the review of systems, ask the closed-ended questions a bit more slowly, pausing occasionally if the patient is thinking about the best response.

Avoid "Right Answer Questions"

Another potential problem with closed questions is what we call the "right answer question." We call it this because it prompts the patient to give the answer the clinician is expecting and probably hoping for. We see it frequently in our workshops during role plays. This is not really a question but rather a kind of confirmation statement. It can be especially dangerous when used with Amiable patients, who are often anxious to please and don't want to upset others. Here are some classic examples: "You're not having any problems with nose bleeds or anything like that?" "No problems sleeping at night?" "No spitting up blood or anything?" "But you haven't noticed any dizziness when you get up quickly?" "But this hasn't happened recently?" Often the clinician's head wags side to side while asking this kind of question, as if saying, "No, none of these problems."

The patient knows what the right answer is! The danger is that the timid or anxious-to-please patient may give the wrong "right" answer. All of these questions would be better phrased as open-ended, or as straightforward closed-ended questions: "What seems to make this worse?" "Have you noticed anything unusual when you blow your nose?" "How are you sleeping at night?" "Do you ever feel dizzy when you suddenly get up?"

When to Use Closed-Ended Questions

We recommend that you use closed-ended questions later in the interview, after you have first used several open-ended questions. Or after using open-ended questions for a while, you can move into a mix of both open and closed queries. The important thing is to use the relationship-establishing open-ended questions first. By then you may have your patient feeling comfortable enough to be cooperative and to maintain a sense of parity even if you do move into using some closed-ended questions.

When to Drop Closed-Ended Questions

A problem we see quite often in our workshops is a clinician asking a perfectly good open-ended question and then immediately closing it up with a related, but closed-ended, question. The beneficial effect of the open-ended "let's-talk" question is suddenly shut off by adding the closed-ended finish.

It sounds like this: "When does it get worse? In the day or at night?" It's better to leave the open-ended part alone and wait for the patient to answer; in other words, "When does it get worse?" (pause).

The patient can give a broad answer to that. But the second, closed-ended question—"In the day or at night?"—closes it up. Suddenly the patient is given an either-or option.

Here's another example of the same thing: "How have you been feeling since I saw you last? Any problem with the medication?" This kind of questioning is such a frequent occurrence that it almost seems that asking open-ended questions is uncomfortable for many clinicians, as if allowing too much control for the patient. When a closed-ended question is added to suddenly shut off the preceding open-ended question, it appears that the clinician is attempting to be conversational but then quickly retreats to the comfortable posture of directing the conversation flow in the I-ask-you-answer, authoritarian mode. When you use a good open-ended question, stop, wait, let it do its work. Don't close it up.

They're Not All Bad

Not every question needs to be rephrased in an open-ended format. For example, "Do you feel pain when I touch here?" or "Does this hurt?" is a useful closed-ended question just as it is, especially helpful during a review of systems. It shouldn't induce passivity in the patient so long as other open-ended questions are also used in the course of the interaction. If you do want to convert the closed-ended question to an open-ended one, ask, for example, "What do you feel when I touch here?"

Some Patients Prefer Closed-Ended Questions

Occasionally a patient may be more comfortable if the session begins with closed-ended questions, especially if she is shy about being there. Starting this way means she can answer and relate with you but doesn't have to perform, feel threatened, or become overwhelmed with the need to talk much. With closed-ended questions, she can just smile and nod at first as you ask, "Are you meeting new people in the retirement home?" "Do you like your new job?" This technique also works well with shy children: "Do you have a favorite teacher?" "Do you have a pet?" Later you can try open questions.

Patients who are from multicultural backgrounds and may be embarrassed because of their limited vocabulary may also prefer having you begin with closed-ended questions, which allows them to start responding to you in the simplest way. As with other shy patients, after they have had a chance to warm up to you and feel comfortable, you can try using open-ended questions with them to obtain more detailed information. Keep in mind that with patients who have limited English, using an interpreter is most desirable. Just because they nod their heads and smile doesn't mean they understand or agree with you.

Switching Quickly Between Open and Closed Questions

Very often the same question can be asked as an open or a closed question. Here is an exercise to give you a sense of how quickly you can switch from closed to open questions. We're not suggesting that you should use only open-ended questions. It's up to you to make the decision when and where to use open or closed questions in the course of a patient interaction. Do you want to encourage the patient to open up? Use open-ended questions. Is it time the patient stopped talking on and on about personal events and focused on the reason for the visit? Use closed-ended questions. This is not guaranteed to change the flow of conversation, but it can influence the degree of talkativeness.

Now that we have looked at various question formats, check how quickly you can rephrase these as open-ended:

1. Did this start recently?

2. Is the pain sharp, or dull?

3. Does it seem to get better when you exercise?

4. Why did you come in today?

5. Did you try aspirin or other medications?

6. Any problem sleeping through the night?

7. Do you understand how you'll be taking the medications?

8. Everything OK at home?

9. Is it mostly on the right side?

10. Are you nervous about this procedure?

11. Have you had this in the past?

12. Where do you feel it most: on the right, or the left?

13. When you get up in the morning, do you feel dizzy?

14. Do you have any other concerns?

15. Do these headaches prevent you from functioning normally on a daily basis?

Here are our answers:

1. When did this start?

2. How would you describe the pain?

3. How does exercise affect this? *or* What happens when you exercise?

4. What brought you in today? *or* How can I help you today?

5. What medications have you tried? *or* What have you tried for this?

6. How are you sleeping? *or* How soundly do you usually sleep at night?

7. This is the question we suggest you restructure, with *you* as the one who wants to check your own clarity of communication. "Just so I'm sure I explained it all clearly, let's go over how you'll be taking the medications."

8. How would you describe the relationships at home? *or* . . . in your family?

9. This is an example of a closed-ended question that is good as is and useful for the review of systems. But if you want to rephrase it as an open-ended question, it would be "Where do you feel it the most?"

10. How are you feeling about this procedure?

11. What's been your experience with this in the past?

12. Drop the closed-ended follow-up question ("on the right or the left"?). Leave it as an open question: "Where do you feel it most?" However, if you want to use it as a closed-ended question, it would be, "Do you feel it more on the right or on the left?"

13. This is actually a closed-ended question, despite the *when* at the beginning. If you want to make it open-ended, you can ask, "What do you notice about your balance when you get up in the morning?"

14. What other concerns do you have about this?

15. What effects do these headaches have on you during the day? or on a daily basis?

Question 13 makes the point that even though *when* is one of the words that typically begin open-ended questions, the phrasing can be misleading. The real beginning of this question is the word *do*: "Do you feel dizzy when you get up in the morning?" The sentence has been inverted so that *when* is only the start of a dependent clause.

USING PROMPTING PHRASES

Another useful technique for eliciting information while showing a caring attitude is through the use of what we call "prompters." These encourage the patient to open up and talk. A prompter can be a simple directive, part of a question, or just one word. If, for example, your patient responds to your question about antibiotics by saying, "I've had bad results with antibiotics," you might say "Such as?" If the patient responds to your information with, "Uh oh! I just *know* what my wife is going to say about this!" you might respond "Which is?" or prompt with "For example?" Such a prodding question fragment, gently spoken and followed by a pause, can be helpful in getting the story from the patient.

Additional prompters are:

- Go on. . . .
- And so . . .
- So you feel . . . ?
- For example . . .
- Tell me about . . .
- In other words . . .
- Let's talk about that more.
- Take me through a typical morning.

The Pause That Reveals

A former colleague and network executive producer enjoys telling the story of TV investigative reporter Mike Wallace being asked, "What's the toughest question you ever asked?" Wallace, he says, replied simply, "My toughest question is, 'And . . . ?'"

Although we certainly don't suggest you use the confrontational style of Mike Wallace when talking with patients, we do support using a question fragment followed by an expectant pause as an effective prompter for getting the real story. Clinicians can also use this combination to gain more information from a patient. Sometimes just a pause alone will do. The wait for a response from your patients may seem interminable, but in all likelihood it's only a few seconds. Try using pauses in your interviews. Even though you have a tight time schedule, your patients probably perceive the time with you as being longer and far more caring if you pause a few beats now and then to wait for their response.

CATCHING EMOTIONAL CLUES

It is important to listen for clues. Some patients avoid speaking openly about their concerns and instead use an oblique, indirect style. Clues might be, "I've just been under so much pressure," or "Oh, I don't know," the latter spoken while looking downward or to the side with a what's-the-use flatness to the voice. Occasionally patients make statements about something that has the potential for being a stronger concern than their manner might imply.

As a communication consultant, I am often asked to observe interactions between clinicians and their patients for later personal coaching. I had occasion to observe rounds in a large Midwestern hospital. Several residents were following the chief of service, a highly respected specialist, brusque and efficient. One dialogue with a patient went like this:

Doctor: Good morning Mrs. Smith. How are you feeling this morning?

Mrs. Smith: Oh, well, not so good.

Doctor: What's bothering you? Did you hold down your breakfast?

Mrs. Smith: I couldn't eat much. I've been kinda worried.

Doctor: Are you sleeping all right?

Mrs. Smith: I don't know. Sorta off and on.

Doctor: Can you sit up pretty well?

Mrs. Smith: I guess. I'm worried, Doctor, that my husband might be acting up, y'know.

Doctor: I see. Were you able to do your physical therapy exercises today?

Mrs. Smith: No I couldn't. I was too upset. My kids are all home alone, and I'm worried about them.

Doctor: Well, don't worry about that. Have you been able to get out of bed at all this morning? Were you able to walk to the bathroom?

Mrs. Smith: Uh-huh.

Doctor: Any trouble walking? Any pain?

Mrs. Smith: (shakes her head no)

Doctor: Well your vitals look good. Your creatinine is up a little, but we won't worry about that just now.

Mrs. Smith: (turning her head on the pillow and looking away) Um-hmm.

Doctor: On the whole, I think you're making pretty good progress, and things are looking good. I'll stop by tomorrow.

He swept hurriedly out the door, followed by five appropriately respectful residents. The young woman who had arranged for me to accompany her stayed behind and said to the patient, "I heard you say you were worried about your husband." A stream of fears poured forth from the distraught patient as she reached out to catch the resident's hand—as if it were a lifeline.

Mrs. Smith's husband, a sometimes violent man, was just out of a thirty-day alcohol treatment program. He was angry with their twelve-year-old son because he had taken the car without permission while Dad was away and put a serious dent in the front fender. The patient was clearly concerned about what might happen while she was away. The resident arranged for a phone to be brought in so the patient could talk with her husband. She was greatly relieved and said to the resident, "That other doctor thought he listened, but he didn't *hear* me. You heard me. That sure means a lot to me, Doctor, and I feel much better now. Thank you."

Take a look at the number of clues the patient drops about her problem that are missed or purposely avoided. Notice the number of times the doctor's response to a psychosocial problem is medical-task-oriented. Jargon is brought in, as if to allay any emotions: "Your vitals look good. Your creatinine is up a little."

Notice also the mismatch in responses. The patient openly expresses herself: "I'm worried. I'm upset." The physician, seeing only from the perspective of the medical task, responds, "I think you're making pretty good progress, and things are looking good." Not to Mrs. Smith, they're not! She finally gives up and turns her head on the pillow, away from the physician.

By vigorously pursuing the information they think will lead to a diagnosis, physicians and other clinicians can miss the clues dropped by patients, who are also seeking empathy. It is not always intended coolness on the part of the clinician. But many patients want more than just medical advice; they also seek empathy and soothing words that will comfort them.

The consequences of not listening carefully to patients can be severe, especially if you gain a reputation in the community for being cold and emotionless; it can contribute to a declining patient pool. Keep in mind that for every patient who complains to you directly, there are probably others who feel the same way but don't tell you.

If patients repeat something or come back to a particular issue later in the interaction, it's probably a clue that they are dropping (Suchman, Markakis, Beckman, and Frankel, 1997). The clues can be subtle but intentional, like Hansel and Gretel's crumbs in the woods, dropped with the hope that you will follow the trail lest they become lost as they go deeper and deeper into the dark forest of their depression or fears.

Here are phrases that indicate a thinly veiled concern—clues that something needs to be followed up:

- "I just don't seem to care anymore."
- "Well, not anymore."
- "I've just been under too much stress lately."
- "Lately I haven't been very interested in . . ."
- "They don't care about me."
- "I'm not looking forward to . . ."
- "Why bother?"

Don't dismiss these phrases as unimportant just because the patient seems to. These hints can often lead you to the real presenting complaint, the deep emotional issue, or even the patient's denial.

On this topic, we should mention that many men—no matter what their personality style—tend to dislike having anything wrong with themselves and may only hint at it, probably in the hope you will pick up the clues and delve deeper into their concerns ("Oh guess I've just been partying a little too much lately" or "Naw, that's just a normal smoker's cough").

Although a patient says, "I've been under a lot of stress lately," it may actually be a case of dealing with a job layoff, an alcoholic spouse, or a teenage child recently into drugs. The patient usually wants you to ferret out what he or she is hinting at. To do so, use open-ended questions and the prompting phrases we covered earlier. It may be the most therapeutic intervention of all.

Stay with the Emotion; Don't Back Away

It was the best role play of the day in a southern California workshop about seven years ago. I was unaware that what we were seeing was actually a drama within a drama. There was a chilling reality about the performance of the role-playing patient, actually a physician in the workshop who had volunteered to be the patient but had not told any of us what the patient's problem was.

Another physician, playing the role of primary care provider, was doing a remarkably skillful job of asking just the right open-ended questions, in just the perfect sequence to bring to light the fact that far more than just a persistent headache had brought the patient in to see him.

Finally the physician leaned slightly forward and asked the patient if he ever thought of harming himself. There was taut silence in the room as the patient sat there, head bowed. Had enough trust between the physician and the patient been established yet? Was there enough of the bonding necessary to ask so profound a question quite this soon? We waited. Silence. Then slowly the patient looked up and replied, "You mean suicide?"

The doctor nodded yes.

Another pause. Then, looking down, the patient responded flatly, "I think about it sometimes." Another heavy pause. "Lots in fact." There it was—his guarded secret. Clearly, the role was a patient who had been covering up his depression.

Suddenly the physician cleared his throat loudly, shifted abruptly in his chair, looked quickly down at the chart, and in a loud voice asked, "Well! Let's see—how's your appetite?"

"Wait a minute!" I called to the physician from the back of the room. "Stay with the emotions here! Don't go abruptly back to the task, business-as-usual, when the patient has just bared his soul to you!"

Another internist disagreed loudly: "But the differential diagnosis! He asked a critical question there. Entirely appropriate when we're dealing with depression. You've *got* to get that!"

"Sure," I agree, "but not at this precise moment."

In such a situation, a troubled patient needs a moment or two of silence, and then perhaps another softly spoken open-ended question to invite him to talk more about his feelings—not asked in a voice dripping with pathos, just a somewhat gentler tone. The physician's suddenly revved-up voice clearly implied, "OK, enough of this emotional stuff. Let's get back to something less embarrassing. Not much I can do about your unmanly emotions. But I can give you some medications for a headache and get you on your way. Straightforward stuff."

The body language was also off. There should have been no uneasy shifting of position in the chair—in fact, no movement at all at such a critical juncture. Certainly no looking down to read the chart, which clearly signaled, "OK. Cut the drama. Let's get back to the data." Even the closed-ended question suggested, "I'll run the show here and get things under control."

So we asked the role-playing patient, "How did you feel when he asked you about your appetite at this point?"

"Kind of abandoned," he said. "I felt like a fool for opening my mouth about it, and probably wouldn't again. We'll just stay on the track and talk about the headaches and what medication or tests might be appropriate. Straightforward stuff."

And this was a fellow physician talking!

Don't Move on Until You Deal with the Emotional Needs

Knowing when to stay with the emotional needs of the patient and when to focus on the medical task is essential. This is not to suggest that the medical task be reduced to secondary importance. We are saying, however, that there is such a thing as critical timing in ordering priorities. This example from a role play clearly illustrates a missed opportunity to bring some empathic listening into an interaction; the clinician returns too quickly to the medical-task questions, which prevents further discussion of the psychosocial issues, which in this case were major.

We later learned that the physician playing the role of the patient had just been through a series of profound losses in his personal life and had been seriously depressed. Fortunately, by the time of the role play he was sufficiently recuperated to be willing to share some of his experiences as well as his insights about dealing in a caring and truly helpful way with those who are seriously depressed.

Lanny lectures nationwide on the topic of depression. He says that the diagnosis of the most common psychosocial disorders, such as depression, anxiety, and drug abuse, is often missed (50–80 percent of the time) because clinicians are not able to pick up the clues from the patient. It's simply inept medicine, he feels, not to establish this diagnosis if the illness of depression is present. Lanny believes it's essential first to make the diagnosis of depression and then to decide whether to treat the patient or refer the patient to another specialist: "Depression accounts for many of the symptoms that patients bring to us. Current studies vary, but it's generally accepted that one out of five women and one out of eight men will have a major depressive episode in their lifetime (Kessler and others, 1994). We absolutely must not miss making this diagnosis if it is present."

Unlock Hidden Concerns

Earlier in this chapter we discussed that one good way to avoid the "Oh, by the way, . . ." is to let the patient talk without interruption or interjected questions at the beginning of the visit. The chief concern then is likely to be revealed earlier in the visit, rather than suddenly surfacing at the end. On a related topic, the main reason for coming to see the clinician may be something other than the patient's presenting complaint in 42 percent of visits, according to researchers. Burack and Carpenter (1983) found that in 96 percent of the cases in which there was a psychosocial problem, what the patient said was the main reason for coming in was not really the principal complaint.

Even when patients' health concerns were largely somatic, the presenting complaint was still not the principal problem in 25 percent of the cases.

This is why we recommend that you make a special effort to use empathic listening and open-ended questions (along with the other listening skills in this chapter) so the patient understands that you are willing to hear his or her psychosocial concerns and are comfortable with discussions of this sort.

If the patient comes to see the clinician because of an unspoken concern and that fear is never brought out and discussed during the visit, the patient either brings it up at the end of the visit or leaves, feeling that an important dimension was missing from the interaction. "Bodily distress by itself seldom brings the patient to the doctor," say Billings and Stoeckle (1989, p. 103) in their excellent textbook *The Clinical Encounter.* "The final extra push to contact a clinician often comes not from the nature of the symptom itself, but from events, called triggers, most of which, surprisingly, are social and psychological rather than biomedical." We believe that an effective way to reveal these triggers is through the use of open-ended questions and responsive listening.

Patients often need signals that you are open to hearing their emotional concerns. Some tip-offs that a patient is struggling with an emotional issue include a voice that breaks, looking downward excessively, sudden prolonged silence, eyes reddening or casting about rapidly, or asking a person who came along to wait outside.

The research of Barbara Korsch, M.D., another widely recognized authority on patient communication, indicates that, particularly in the pediatric setting, if the patient is not able to discuss the emotional component there is less satisfaction with the encounter (Korsch, Gozzi, and Francis, 1968). Despite this, less than 10 percent of all the talk during a medical visit is devoted to psychosocial topics, including questions and counseling (Bertakis, Roter, and Putnam, 1991).

Open-Ended Questions: The Key to Unlocking Secrets

Deep-seated emotional problems are seldom coaxed out by means of closed-ended questions. The key to opening up hidden concerns is the

Communicating with Today's Patient

open-ended question ("What other concerns do you have?"). Avoid the type of closed question we previously described: "Any other problems?" It's just too easy for the amiable patient to say "Oh no" and smile agreeably. Or you might use a prompter and say, "It would help me to know what other questions or concerns you might have."

Many clinicians hesitate to ask this type of question, fearing it might open up another ten minutes of questions and answers. But it can actually be more effective and efficient to deal with these issues at this point in the visit, not in the final seconds—and that can save you time in the long run. We often see articles on patient communication that suggest you ask this question at the end of the visit, but we strongly recommend that you ask it during the history to save time, get a better diagnosis, and avoid last-minute concerns.

OTHER IMPORTANT TECHNIQUES TO ENHANCE PSYCHOSOCIAL COMMUNICATION

These are simply ways that you can encourage your patients to open up their hidden fears and let them know you are willing to hear their psychosocial issues.

Maintain Good Eye Contact

As the patient begins to confide emotional concerns, be sure to look the patient in the eye, signaling that you are not backing off from the emotion and will stay with the patient, helping however you can. In a study by van Dulmen and her team of researchers, the more the physician looked at the patient, the more psychosocial information was delivered (van Dulmen, Verhaak, and Bilo, 1997).

Remove Barriers

Consider taking off your glasses if your patient begins to tell you something that is deeply emotional, as we mentioned in Chapter Four on body language. It removes a barrier between you. It's as if you are symbolically exchanging your "thinking apparatus" for some person-to-person sharing with unhindered eye contact in order to have an intimate, humanistic conversation with your patient. This can be done in an entirely professional manner. Be sure also to keep the rest of your body language open, with nothing blocking the front of the chest, such as folded arms or clutched charts.

Stop Moving

Keep all movements to a minimum if the patient begins to tell you something deeply emotional. This is not the time to write in the chart or do any other medical task. You can do that a bit later. Stay with the feeling. The patient will usually perceive you as caring and feel that you are spending more time than you actually are.

Slow Down Your Speech

Slow your speech and soften your voice somewhat when asking difficult questions or those with a psychosocial aspect. This should done subtly and professionally rather than making them abrupt or obvious. But a loud, assertive, staccato voice pattern is not as inviting as a slow, modulated voice that encourages the patient to openly discuss his emotional issues. Try drawing out your vowels a bit more during these moments.

Save the Toughest Questions for Later

You are likely to get good, complete answers to questions that are potentially embarrassing if you ask them later in the interview, after your patient has gained a sense of comfort and trust with you. Questions about bodily functions, sexual habits or sexual performance, use of alcohol or drugs, and the like are more likely to be answered candidly when the patient feels safe and cared for. If possible, save the tougher questions until after you've softened the environment by taking a sincere, personal interest in patients and by commiserating with their difficulties, if only through body language.

Check Back Later

If you ask a question that is important and the patient does not answer or you suspect he is withholding essential information, you can drop the issue and return to it later. When you come back to the question, be sure to use different, perhaps simpler, words on rephrasing. And stay with open-ended questions. As we said, that's what opens up patient secrets. Closed-ended questions are too easy to wiggle out of answering.

Verbally Review the Patient's Chief Concerns

After gathering the information you need during the history, repeat the patient's stated concerns. Repeating the main problems tells patients you listened and you consider their concerns important. It also gives the patient a chance to think about bringing up any other issues that might be difficult to discuss.

Probe Further for Hidden Concerns

After the patient tells you the chief concern, gently probe a little further, to discover whether the patient has more concerns that are being hidden. Avoid the word *problems,* as in, "Any other problems?" Those who have the style of the Amiable patient tend to avoid bothering you with "problems" but might be willing to reveal "concerns." Then you might ask, "What else did you want to bring to my attention today?" This open-ended question is more inviting than just a closed, "Anything else?"

Speaking of the Amiable patient, this is the social style most likely to harbor hidden concerns. As we said in Chapter Three on social styles, it's less likely to be Driving or Expressive patients who keep things hidden. People with these styles are more likely to tell you straight out what's bothering them. Those with the Amiable traits are less comfortable telling you anything they think might upset you or take up too much of your valuable time.

Whatever your patient's social style, take those few moments to connect. If the patient senses that you're listening in a way that shows you sincerely care, your patient is more likely to open up to you. And that's when you can get the unique story of the illness, what it means, and how it presents in that particular patient.

By using the listening techniques we've covered here, you'll have your accurate diagnosis, probably in less time—and you'll cement your relationship with the patient for years to come.

Now that we have the diagnosis, the treatment regimen needs to be explained to the patient. In the next chapter, we look at some communication techniques that help your patients understand your prescribed therapy and also encourage them to follow your recommendations.

CHAPTER 6

Explanations Patients Can Understand and Remember

"Your angiogram is scheduled for next week," the cardiologist begins. He is explaining to his nervous patient what the upcoming test entails. Leaning back in a relaxed position, he casually continues, "Well . . . basically, we just force a tube into your heart, shoot you with radioactive dye, and light up your vessels."

This scene is from a role play in a recent patient communication workshop.

"Is that how you tell *all* your patients about angiograms?" I gasped. "That's about it," he replied with a shrug of his shoulders. *How many patients actually come back to have the procedure?* I started to ask, and then figured I probably knew.

EXPLANATIONS THAT GET THE RESULTS YOU WANT

In this chapter, we build on previous chapters and look at techniques that enhance explanations, specifically addressing two goals: (1) how to give explanations so patients understand the information before leaving your office and (2) how to explain so that they act on your recommendations.

The original meaning of the word *doctor* is "teacher," from the Latin *docere*, to teach. Whether you are a physician, physician assistant, nurse practitioner, or another type of health care professional, the primary way you teach patients is by giving them clear explanations. Educating your patients is an important medical task that is based on solid scientific foundations.

Physicians generally spend about 25 percent of their time in the office—four minutes out of every fifteen-minute patient visit—giving information, instructing, and counseling (Grüninger, 1995). You probably give between fifty and a hundred explanations every day: about treatment plans, medications, surgical procedures, directions to an office, how the referral process works, covered benefits—the list seems to get longer each year. But in today's time crunch, it's easy to foreshorten medical explanations, or to quickly wrap up the session with a terse, "Call if you have any questions" or "Check with the nurse if you need to go over anything again."

Risk Management

Although we touched on this point earlier, it bears repeating here, since it is strongly tied to explanations. Looking into what specific behaviors were associated with lessening the risk of malpractice, a team of researchers found that physicians with no malpractice claims educated their patients more often about what to expect during a test or first visit. They also used more humor, gave more encouragement, and asked about patients' opinions and understanding of their situation more often than did physicians who had a history of claims (Levinson and others, 1997). The time spent educating your patients can also have the effect of reinforcing your relationship with them, a relationship of trust and loyalty—another of the many "two for the price of one" benefits derived from clear, thorough explanations.

Shared Decision Making

In nine out of ten decisions researchers found that physicians in office practice did not sufficiently discuss the issues involved so that the patient could make an informed choice. The decisions were in three categories: basic (e.g., routine lab tests), intermediate (e.g., medication issues), and complex (e.g., prostate cancer screening). None of the intermediate decisions and only 0.5 percent of the complex decisions met the criteria for completeness of informed consent (Braddock and others, 1999).

What Patients Want to Know About Their Illness

Patients want to know certain basics about their illness, certainly the name of the illness and a description of it. They also want to know what's ahead, and whether it will get worse. They are often concerned about how their illness will affect their life and how they can cope with it. Patients also want to know about the treatment plan and how it will fit into their life. Sometimes they want to know what caused their illness. To help them understand all this, patients want understandable and thorough explanations that don't confuse, terrify, or overwhelm them—as the cardiologist's explanation of the angiogram surely would.

Why Patients Misunderstand or Don't Listen to Explanations

Six hundred physicians and other clinicians who attended Desmond Medical Communications workshops over a six-year period were asked, by questionnaire, why they thought patients sometimes misunderstood explanations. Two hundred forty-seven respondents, the majority of whom were family practice physicians or internists, gave patients' "denial of their situation" as the main reason. Another 215 respondents cited patients' "lack of health education," making it the second most commonly perceived cause of misunderstanding. Pediatricians reversed the two, citing lack of health education as the chief reason (DeFleur and Desmond, forthcoming).

Another reason for patients' misunderstandings may be that sometimes physicians' explanations are not as clear as they might be. To a physician or other clinician, it makes perfect sense to say, "I recommend this medication regimen because, left untreated, your hypertension could increase your risk of renal failure, myocardial infarction, and cerebral hemorrhage." It would make absolutely no sense at all, however, to large numbers of patients, leaving them more befuddled than motivated to comply with the clinician's recommendations.

When the physicians and other health care professionals were asked on the questionnaire why they thought patients didn't listen, they gave "lack of attention/do not want to listen" as the major reason (46 percent), which did not vary much over the period from 1993 to 1998. The second most frequent response was that patients were vague or disoriented, which was a fairly steady 20 percent over the six-year period. Only 3 percent said patients didn't listen due to hearing loss or deafness. So the task seems to be to deliver information in a such a way that the patient will want to pay attention and listen.

The word *communicate* means to give to another as a partaker, to exchange thoughts. The original Latin word means to share. This implies not doing all the talking, checking for understanding, and encouraging an open exchange of ideas. The techniques we cover in this chapter, as well as those in the previous chapter on listening, offer a number of ways to do that.

The Advantages of Taking Time to Explain

Even though the time for consultations seems squeezed to the limit, taking the time to give clear explanations greatly benefits your patients, and you as well. Patient education has a clearly proven impact on health outcomes, including reducing morbidity and even mortality (Mazzuca, 1982). Patients who take an active role, ask questions, and become knowledgeable about their illness seem to do better. In fact, they do significantly better than patients who remain passive and less knowledgeable (Kaplan, Greenfield, and Ware, 1989).

Patients who are given more information tend to be satisfied with the visit and tend to remember and understand the information better. They are also more likely to follow your instructions and to adhere to the medications or treatment plans you prescribe (Hall, Roter, and Katz, 1988). When patients fully understand and agree with your recommendations, those patients are likely to follow your advice and, as a result, have better health outcomes (Carter, Inui, Kukull, and Haigh, 1982).

CLEAR EXPLANATIONS SAVE TIME

If a patient leaves your office unclear about important aspects of the illness or treatment regimen, the result can be a return visit or a telephone call from the patient or a family member asking you for clarification. In a worst-case situation, the patient fails to improve because of not understanding how to follow your treatment recommendations accurately. Or the patient switches to another medication out of frustration—a medication that may not be indicated.

All these scenarios cause stress and dissatisfaction for the patient and for you, as well as affecting the medical outcomes. They all mean considerable loss of time and are far more costly for you both.

Patients Lodge Fewer Complaints

In terms of patient satisfaction, one of the most frequent patient complaints I see in many of my clients' customer-satisfaction surveys is, "Didn't understand what the doctor said. I want clearer explanations!" How many hours does it take for you to deal with a single patient complaint lodged because of a perceived poor explanation? "Physicians who give clear explanations to their patients are likely to be seen as competent and caring. In turn, these patient perceptions may have a profound effect on the relationship between the clinician and the patient and on the entire course of illness" (Roter and Hall, 1992, p. 13).

Patients Ask Fewer Last-Minute Questions

If patients are given thorough information about the therapeutic regimen, they are less apt to raise new questions at the end of the visit, according to a number of studies (see for example White, Levinson, and Roter, 1994). Giving full explanations can include using plastic models, pictures, or other visual aids, and handing out pamphlets or brochures as supplemental explanation material. Throughout this chapter, you'll find a variety of useful tips and techniques for giving patients thorough yet understandable information— suggestions that take into consideration your time constraints.

EDUCATING THE PATIENT THROUGH EXPLANATIONS

Because patients who are more knowledgeable about their illness are more likely to follow your instructions and feel satisfied with your care, here are some approaches you can use to educate your patients.

Narrate During the Exam

It's more interesting to patients if you narrate occasionally as you examine them. It's also an opportunity to educate the patient. For example, you might tell a patient what you are checking as you palpate an area—without alarming him, of course. "This is where your pancreas is. Now let's check in the area of your stomach. Do you feel anything as I press here? OK." and so forth. It helps the patient better understand what is happening, and it documents your thoroughness—more so than if you remain silent and don't share information until the exam is over.

With intermittent narration, the patient is brought into the process and subtly encouraged to assume a role of partnership with you. In an era when we want patients to be more responsible for their health, narrating from time to time during the exam can be a way of inviting patients to be actively involved—to become knowledgeable and surveillant about their own health. If patients lie there passively during your exam, they can feel left out of the loop or intimidated by the unknown. ("Uh-oh. I wonder why she went over that spot again. Is there something really wrong there?") The opportunity is ripe for fearing the worst, which is why many people avoid going to the clinic to be checked out in the first place.

When the Patient Is in the Dark

"Patients are just too demanding today!" a physician assistant complained in a recent workshop, quickly citing an example. He had given a standard neurological exam to a young woman who came in with a recent-onset headache. The test results were normal, but she was not satisfied and insisted on an x-ray to find out "what was wrong inside her head." I asked him if he had narrated during the neurological exam. He had not.

Communicating with Today's Patient

His patient's dissatisfaction may have emanated largely from the seeming simplicity of the basic neuro exam and her lack of understanding or appreciation of its validity. In our high-tech era, the standard neuro exam can seem pretty low-tech to many patients. If the physician assistant had told the young woman what he was checking for as he went through the exam—holding a pencil vertically in front of her eyes, tapping her knee, and so forth—it might have given her more confidence in this test.

He could have explained the importance of the neurological exam—that it can give valuable and essential information, including information needed to rule out a number of possible causes of her headache, which helps the clinician formulate the proper diagnosis.

Explaining the importance of the neurological exam and narrating during the exam might have left the patient feeling better about the test. Instead, she questioned the quality of care and the caregiver.

You've probably guessed the rest of the story. The patient complained loudly to the patient representative and to other administrators and was able to get her x-ray—and a new primary care clinician.

It could have been a different story. Explaining why the exam is effective and narrating occasionally ("now I'm checking your reflexes," and so forth) wouldn't have taken any more time—certainly less time than it took to wrangle with the patient representative over the situation. The clinician might have learned more about the patient's health beliefs, providing yet another opportunity to educate the patient—in this case, that x-rays don't just "look inside your head." It might have spared the patient unnecessary exposure to x-rays, avoided the utilization costs involved, and prevented the bad feelings evoked all around.

In addition, the patient might still be in the fold. The seeds of uncertainty and doubt in the patient's mind often grow into negative feelings and ultimately lack of confidence in the caregiver.

Using Analogies and Similes

Analogies or similes that are appropriate can be a very graphic way to give an explanation to patients in terms they can understand or visualize. An internist on the television medical talk show I hosted used a garden hose to explain high blood pressure: "What happens to the blood vessels when you have high blood pressure can be compared to using a garden hose. If you turn on the water full force and then pinch the hose, the pressure inside the hose will build up. Over time that pressure could weaken the walls of the hose. That's somewhat similar to what can happen to your blood vessels when your blood pressure is too high."

If the medical concepts are complex, an analogy or simile can simplify them and bring the patient a sense of understanding and involvement. Family physician Terry Ruhl actively encourages this use of analogies in giving explanation. One of his favorites: "Your blood is like a river, carrying things from one place to another. Oxygen from the air you breathe gets carried in special barges called red blood cells. If you don't have enough of these barges, you can't carry enough oxygen. Your iron pills are letting your body build more red blood cells, or barges" (Ruhl, 1999, p. 2). He warns, however, that misconceptions can arise from the use of analogies, so once the basic idea—or target concept—is learned, the patient needs to be weaned from the analogy by further explanation of the situation.

An analogy can be used to explain why one diagnostic test is preferred over another at a particular point. For example, if a patient wants a CT scan for her headaches, which began only recently, you might say something like this:

Well, yes, we could use a CT scan to look for possible causes for your headaches. At this point, however, a CT scan would be a little like taking a jetliner to go to the corner grocery. It would really be faster and easier to walk there or drive your car. In a similar way, we generally start out with some very good tests that give us the important information that we need to have at this point in our investigation of your headaches. Another advantage of these tests is that they're also easier for you to take, and we can get those test results faster than if we schedule you for a CT scan.

We recommend that you add, "But if we find that you *do* need to have a CT scan later, to give us additional information, that's certainly what you'll have."

Use Other Figures of Speech as Needed

It's important of course, that any analogies, similes, or other figures of speech that you use align clearly with the situation you are trying to simplify. If used appropriately with the medical message, figures of speech can be very powerful aids to educating your patients.

A favorite phrase of Lanny's is "tincture of time." It can be used, for example, after you have your findings, have suggested a treatment plan, and believe that no further tests are indicated at this time. You might want to add words to this effect: "Often a 'tincture of time' helps tell us whether we need to do more studies. So, let's see you again in three weeks and check on how you're doing." It lends a certain warmth and continuity of care to the fact that you do not think more tests are in order at this time.

In the pediatric setting, figures of speech may make your explanations easier for a child to understand, especially if they draw clearly on what is already familiar to the child. Lanny has a delightful technique he uses with children who need to have their throats looked at. He takes a tongue depressor and quickly draws a face and body on it, telling his young patients that this is a stick man and they can take the stick man home with them. Then he tells them he has another stick man who wants to look down their throat. They open wide—usually with a smile on their tiny faces.

When Simple Metaphors Go Awry

Problems can arise with everyday words if they are "hidden metaphors": words and phrases we use frequently without even thinking of them as being simple metaphors. These can be easily misconstrued, or taken too literally by some patients, particularly by children.

In the Pediatric Population. Marie, age four, had been in with her mother to see the pediatrician for her allergies. Marie's mother was given an inhaler with the instruction to have Marie use it at night. "It'll open up her chest," the pediatrician explained, "and help her breathe more freely." That night, when Marie began to wheeze, her mother brought out the inhaler. Marie screamed in terror. "What's the matter?" her concerned mother asked. But Marie only huddled beneath the blankets and refused the inhaler. Finally, she was coaxed into trying it just once. "Mommy," she sobbed, still trembling, "Will I bleed all over?" Her mother looked puzzled and asked Marie why she thought she'd "bleed all over." "When . . . when this opens up my chest," the frightened child whispered in terror. Words and concepts that an adult can easily put into context may cause problems for the young child who takes them literally.

If you address your explanations, in part at least, to the child rather than the parent, this may help you remember to focus on using easy-to-understand language.

In the Foreign-Born Population. When English is the patients' second language, it can be especially important to avoid using colloquialisms and hidden metaphors. They may be taken too literally or have a different meaning for the patient. For example, a nurse practitioner discussing her patient's diet added in a lighter vein: "Well, sometimes the flesh is willing but the spirit is a little weak." The patient, recently arrived from Russia, thought she meant, "Meat is OK for you, but vodka needs to be watered down."

When Patients Come with Their Own Metaphors. Sometimes patients come in with their own metaphors and analogies about medical topics. Researchers in Denmark found that because patients often don't understand all aspects of the scientific explanation of a disease, they tend to fall back on their own experiences—or their own imaginative resources—to make sense of the explanation. If a clinician tries to draw a patient radically away from these resources for conceptualizing, it can cause serious confusion or even a breakdown in the communication effort (Mabeck and Olesen, 1997). So it might be better to work with your patient's concepts—or gently tweak them as necessary—but avoid throwing them out altogether. Here again, you might need to wean the patient gently away from the metaphorical concept by means of further education and an easy-to-understand explanation.

Using Statistics

Many health care attorneys prefer to see clinicians use statistics in their explanations rather than metaphors, analogies, or other figures of speech. When a patient asks about one treatment approach over another, for example, many attorneys recommend using a statistic to explain whenever possible. This recommendation is largely because if a metaphor or analogy is used inappropriately, the patient is left with the wrong impression and the result could be misunderstandings or unrealistic expectations leading to lawsuits.

For example, you could say, "Although I can't guarantee a perfect outcome, I can tell you that in 80 percent of the cases—or in eight out of ten patients who have this procedure—the results are good." You might add, "And we certainly hope you will be among that 80 percent who have positive results, Mr. Gonzales!" This is preferable, some attorneys tell us, to analogies such as, "You're safer having this procedure done than you are when you get on the local freeway and drive to the other side of town." But the latter certainly has more impact, especially if it is statistically accurate. If you think your patient will benefit from a well–thought-out and basically accurate metaphor or simile, we suggest you use it, keeping the attorneys' caveat in mind.

Instead of talking in terms of "80 percent of cases," you'll notice in this example we add "eight out of ten patients." That has much more impact because it has a human connection and is more likely to be remembered since it talks about people instead of "cases." Patients can more readily visualize and identify with another patient, or even numbers of other patients, than with percentages. For example, "One out of eight women will get breast cancer" is more likely to be remembered by the patient you are encouraging to examine her breasts monthly than "breast cancer occurs in 12.5 percent of the female population."

Handouts Can Supplement Your Explanation

When patients are diagnosed, they're usually given a lot of new information verbally by their clinician. Already worried and probably not feeling well, many patients find this verbal presentation of new information about what's happening to them and what their treatment may entail rather hard to follow and even harder to remember.

In addition to your own explanation, consider giving patients an educational handout about their particular problem, whether it's a gallbladder, prostate cancer, or backache problem. The brochures reinforce the information you give them during the office visit and help clarify any confusion they might have about their condition once they get home. Brochures and handouts can also be a handy resource for answering the questions family members or friends may have regarding the diagnosis and prognosis. Keep patient handouts in the examination room so you have easy access to them. These are used only as a supplement to your own thorough explanation, of course.

Customize and Personalize Handouts. Instead of just handing the patient a brochure or pamphlet, give it a personal touch and write the patient's name on it, perhaps at the top. You can customize it even further by checking or circling information that is particularly pertinent for that patient. This only takes a few seconds and can be done while you are talking or explaining something further. But it sends the message that the patient is getting more than just your standard handout—something customized especially for him or her.

Handouts from Your Computer. Many resources for patient education handouts are available through the Internet. These materials can be quickly printed out from your computer to give to the patient during the office visit. Some of these Internet resources even allow you to print the patient's name on the handout.

We strongly recommend that even if the computer added the patient's name, you still need to personalize it with your own writing. Jot a few personal comments on the handout, such as, "Especially important . . ." or "Please note . . ." We also suggest you check, circle, or underline text that you want the patient to pay particular attention to—not only because you want the patient to read the handout but also because you're adding a warm, personal touch to customize this high-tech information. Add your name and perhaps the patient's name, as we suggested earlier.

When to Avoid Customizing Handouts. There are a few instances when writing the patient's name—or yours—on the handout can jeopardize patient confidentiality. For example, if an HIV handout is inadvertently left on a coffee shop counter, or an Alcoholics Anonymous brochure drops out of a pocket, it's better if no patient names are on them.

Draw Pictures

Studies have shown that on average people remember about 20 percent of what they hear and 40 percent of what they see, but a full 70 percent of what they see *and* hear (Rouwenhorst, 1996). Patients generally like the diagrams or illustrations you make to clarify where a certain organ is located or what will be done during surgery, not only because it helps them understand the situation better but also because the drawings or diagrams you make for them are individualized ("This is *my* gallbladder"). It's more personal and customized than the three-color professional illustration of the gallbladder that you keep in your office to show all your gallbladder patients. Based on our informal surveys of both physicians and patients, we've learned that patients tend to put these hand-drawn illustrations on the refrigerator or medicine cabinet at home, or keep them in their wallet to whip out for interested friends and relatives to see.

Of course, drawings and diagrams rendered too hastily or inaccurately can have dire results. A surgeon we know tried to convey to his patient, who spoke very little English, where he would be making the incision during the man's upcoming abdominal surgery. He drew a stick figure on a small piece of paper and then, to indicate where he would make the incision, he ripped the paper in half. The patient fled in terror and never returned. Had the surgeon rendered a full torso, then carefully drawn the smaller incision area, he might have performed the surgery.

Keep Writing Pads Handy

Keep small tablets of paper in each exam room. Ideally, such pads have your name or the clinic name, or both, printed at the top. These notepads are very handy for writing down instructions and for drawing pictures.

We have been surprised over the years to hear many clinicians tell us they use their prescription pads to render drawings or diagrams for patients, jot down foods to avoid eating, make reminders on how to desensitize an allergy patient's bedroom, and even record the phone number or address of the referral physician. Some clinicians have told us they occasionally tear off a piece of the paper covering the exam table to make these notes for patients!

Neither prescription pads nor exam table paper is an acceptable alternative; notepads of whatever size you think appropriate should be in your room, or perhaps in your pocket if you change rooms frequently during the day. Using your prescription pads to write instructions or jot the name of an over-the-counter medication is dangerous, since some patients or their relatives can rewrite the prescription to obtain illegal drugs.

Having small pads printed can be inexpensive. Next time you have prescription pads printed, say a thousand or so, have another thousand printed for notepads; it will be at only a small extra charge. Be sure to ask the printer to delete the Rx, your DEA number, any extra lines on the pad, or whatever else you want to have deleted. You will then have your thousand prescription pads plus a thousand notepads with a professional header, all for a considerable savings over having notepads alone printed.

Use Other Visual Aids

People have different ways of reacting to information giving, as we discussed in Chapter Three. Some like charts, graphs, and statistics, and others respond best to visual stimuli. However, plastic models of knee joints, ear canals, and other models of body parts can help most patients under-

Communicating with Today's Patient

stand and remember what is involved in their own illness. We also like using automatic slide shows and videotapes that patients can watch to learn more about their condition and how to cope with it.

HOW BODY LANGUAGE AFFECTS EXPLANATIONS

Body language factors into how well your explanation is received by a patient. It can significantly reinforce your message or say something entirely different.

Focus on Important Points with Eye Contact

Be sure to look at your patients whenever you make key points in your explanations to them. This heightens the importance of your words; patients are likely to listen more carefully and give the information higher priority.

Where You Sit Sets the Stage for Understanding

You can further enhance your explanation and at the same time send the silent, implied message, via body language, that you are encouraging patients to take an active role in their own health care by simply moving your chair or stool next to the patient. You wheel around so that you are sitting side by side with the patient. The test results or other information is in front of you both: "In looking at this angiogram, we can see that the main artery that supplies the heart with blood, here, is partially blocked. . . ." The patient will have a clearer understanding and will feel more enfranchised in the process if you are on the same side of the table. Whether you are reviewing a treatment plan with the patient, going over an informed consent statement, or giving any other kind of explanation, this side-by-side position sets up a team dynamic and enhances understanding. It also implies that you respect the patient and welcome that patient's input and involvement.

When role-play patients in our workshop (actually clinicians who volunteer for the task) are asked what difference they feel in being side by side rather than opposite the clinician, they always respond that they feel more involved and usually say they feel more comfortable about their relationship with the caregiver.

"Finding" the Right Word

The venerable phrase "do no harm" extends to the language you use as well as to other medical interventions available to you. Some medical terms routinely used with patients who have chronic diseases are actually quite hurtful: "Well, since you have this degree of abnormality . . ." or "This is what we call boutonnière deformity." Hearing terms of this sort often leaves these patients feeling depressed and deformed.

Instructors in the Arthritis Educator Program at the University of Texas's Southwestern Medical Center at Dallas prefer to use the noun *finding*. As they instruct physicians and other health care professionals on how to conduct a musculoskeletal examination, they also encourage the clinicians to use this word and other nonhurtful terms when talking with their patients. The arthritis educators understand firsthand how important it is to use language that is not discouraging or depressing, since they have arthritis themselves. Instead of saying, "When you have this level of deformity in your feet, you have to . . ." say, "When we have a finding of this sort in the major joints of the foot, then I recommend. . . ." Although it may not be possible to avoid the conventional terms all the time, we recommend you try to use a less painful version whenever you can. Here is a list of preferable words to replace the commonly used medical terms that can leave patients feeling discouraged or depressed:

Hurtful Term	Preferable Term
Disfigurement	Alignment, finding, situation, condition
Deformity	Alignment, finding, situation, condition
Abnormality	Changes, findings
Complaint	Concern
Crippled	Condition, situation
Handicap	Situation, condition
Problem	Concern, situation
Degenerative disease	This condition
End-stage	At this point, now

A colleague with rheumatoid arthritis who had just undergone surgical fusion of her ankle asked her primary care physician whether she could wear higher-heeled shoes for special occasions. He shot back: "You rheumatoids just aren't willing to accept reality! You're going to limp the rest of your life. Deal with it!" This intelligent, attractive, professional woman quickly dealt with his rudeness; she found someone else to oversee her routine care.

Avoid Information Overload

Try not to cluster many units of information in one sentence. As you are explaining something important, build a few pauses into your flow of words to allow the patient time to grasp the information.

Jargon is often the culprit in information overload, so let's take a closer look at it in the next section.

JARGON: ITS USES AND ABUSES

On the TV talk show "Doctors' House Call," which I hosted a few years ago, a viewer called in, perplexed: "My doctor says I need angioplasty, and I don't understand why." The guest cardiologist on the show responded, "Well, when coronary angiography reveals severe obstruction in the coronary arteries, then percutaneous transluminal coronary angioplasty may be indicated. Does that answer your question?"

Suddenly a loud disconnect buzz was sounded as the telephone line went dead. All the viewers knew she'd hung up! It was almost like a comedy routine from "Saturday Night Live." The viewer had probably switched to CNN—where they speak English.

Our TV program was clearly in trouble, as viewers continued to drift away each week. Even though this was an opportunity to ask questions of physicians and other health care professionals on a variety of topics, people weren't calling in, and few even watched. I suggested one of our workshops in media training for the physicians who were scheduled to be on all future programs.

The results of these workshops were immediate. As the clinicians appeared on the programs using their new communication skills, viewers began calling in again. In fact, in the weeks that followed, the clinicians had to stay in the TV studio an extra hour to answer the overflow of telephone calls still coming in from viewers even after we were no longer on air.

In our next season, "Doctors' House Call" won the national CableACE Award for excellence in a program series. The judges said the doctors seemed very approachable and helpful. The main goals of the media training workshops had been to help the clinicians reduce jargon and give clear, easy-to-understand explanations. Our shiny silver CableACE Award testifies that understandable, approachable clinicians do have mass appeal.

A Foreign Language

Medical terminology is said to have a vocabulary that is equivalent to two complete foreign languages. Confronted with any foreign language, most of us try to guess at what the foreign words mean. You probably did this the last time you visited a place where English is not the primary language spoken. We say to ourselves, "Sounds like . . ." and do our best to guess what the word means. So do patients.

Some malapropisms have become classics of medical humor. You may have seen or even own T-shirts with such garbled medical terms and amusing translations of jargon as these:

- Idiopathic: low intelligence
- Ambulatory: come in by ambulance
- Atrophy: there'll be a prize
- Congenital: you're friendly
- Etiology: the study of eating

And so forth.

The language of medical acronyms has grown recently to become yet another foreign language to most patients. The alphabet soup served up in health care today is often hard to digest and draws more patient complaints than hospital food: "Mrs. Jones, the OB-GYN your PCP referred you to has ordered a SMAC and an MRI. We're going to draw the SMAC today—provided you've been NPO. But, the HMOs and PPOs require that the MRI be approved at PCC. The HPC will call you with the decision, but just call the MIC in the managed care department if you have any questions. OK?"

There are even veteran health care professionals out there who don't understand what all that means. It illustrates how essential it is to break this kind of medicalese down into bite-sized, easily digestible pieces of information.

It's unsettling when we can't understand what someone is saying, when we can't quite get it. We feel befuddled, stupid, or angry. Patients have a variety of reactions when they hear jargon used. If their reaction is negative, it can affect your relationship. It can also cut you off from a primary source of information about the patient's ailment: the patient.

If you give an explanation heavily infused with jargon and then ask, "Is that clear?" or "Do you understand how you'll be taking your medications?" few patients will say, "Gee no, I just didn't get it, Dr. Smith. Could you go through it all again—slowly?" More likely when you ask if they understand, patients will smile and nod, seeming to understand. But too many go home not at all clear about what to do. In communications, we often say, "The measure of whether you communicated effectively is determined by the results you get." If a patient doesn't understand, it's often due to the communication techniques used in explaining.

Why Don't They Listen?!

Jargon connotes a difference in status and therefore encourages passivity in some patients. You've probably dealt with patients who seem to be afraid to ask questions even though they need to better understand their disease and its treatment. Sometimes they may not want to hear the answer because of their own denial or fear, but another reason may be that you and the medical setting intimidate them. Add jargon into the mix, and they can be completely overwhelmed, quickly retreating into passivity:

"This whole thing is way too complicated. I'll just leave everything up to the doctor."

Some people have suggested that's just what many clinicians want: a quiet, passive patient who won't take up time with lots of questions. But as we pointed out earlier, patients who are knowledgeable and stay actively involved in their own health care tend to fare better in a shorter amount of time than do patients who remain passive.

Jargon can cause resentment in some patients. They feel angry when they hear polysyllabic medical terms, perceiving the speaker as showing off or trying to sound superior. To them it sounds patronizing and thereby distances you from them.

And some like it! There are patients who actually prefer having your explanations peppered with medical terms, since they connect it to your knowledge base and consider it a measure of your expertise. Some patients even perceive it as a compliment to them, indicating your awareness that they are also highly educated and capable of understanding those terms.

Although using jargon gets a lot of bad press, it's really a mixed bag in terms of patient preferences and in terms of appropriateness. How can you best deal with jargon? Here are some suggestions.

Jargon Can Be Useful for Special Patients. There are times when medical jargon is entirely appropriate. It can be necessary, for example, with certain patients who have chronic illnesses and are likely to hear the same medical terms used frequently during their treatment, such as *autoimmune, subluxation,* or *platelets.* The medical terms may offer an opportunity to educate these chronic patients about their diseases. Jargon can also be useful as a medical shorthand—a quick way to communicate if patients are already educated about their illness when you see them.

Make Jargon Understandable. Use the simple, easy-to-understand term first, followed by the medical term. Avoid the reverse order, giving the more complicated medical term first. This can lead to information overload and a shutting down of attention.

Use a "bridging" phrase, such as "or as we call it": "We need to have special x-rays of the heart, or what we refer to in medical terms as an angiogram." That approach can help educate patients without overwhelming them with polysyllabic words.

One rheumatologist told us that, during patient exams, he routinely used to utter phrases such as, "I see your metacarpalphalangeal joints are erthyenemous, with active synovial involvement." Now, he says he begins with simple phrases, such as "It must be hard to get your ring off," and then continues with the explanation about joint swelling, using simple, clear language: "That's because right here at this joint . . ." and so on.

When to use jargon is a judgment call; it depends on the patient's education and background and your perception of the patient's ability to understand the medical information.

Say It Again, in a Different Way

In her research on patient interactions, Barbara Korsch found that when patients didn't seem to understand, physicians would often just repeat their words again and again (Korsch, Gozzi, and Francis, 1968). I have noticed a similar phenomenon, except that frequently the clinician not only repeats the same words over and over but says them louder! Use different and certainly simpler words when you rephrase your explanations.

When Bad Is Positive and Good Is Negative

If you tell a patient her stress test was positive, she might sigh with relief. *Positive* to most laypeople is a good thing, and many don't realize that in medicine it can be bad news (though common use of "HIV-positive" has gone a long way to counter that idea). Conversely, the patient may frown and be fearful if you report that a test came back negative.

What is even more confusing to many patients is the term *false positive*. It sounds like a "no-yes," and the term always bears explaining unless your patient is experienced with medical testing and understands this term.

All Patients Are Remarkable. The patient is a young professional woman, sitting on the exam table, disrobed, feeling chilly and a bit foolish. The physician walks in to meet his new patient. After glancing over her chart, he looks at her as she sits there, shivering in her plain paper wrapper, and then comments, "From what I see, you're pretty unremarkable." Unremarkable! Everyone likes to think they are remarkable. Many patients don't understand that it can be a good thing to hear a clinician say those words.

Avoid using *unremarkable* in talking about patients, whether you are addressing them directly or even indirectly—as you dictate notes or talk with colleagues in the hall. *Unremarkable* to the rest of the world means not worthy of notice and connotes that the patient is of no interest, of little value. In this case, the patient was so infuriated she not only changed physicians but also wrote up the incident in her professional association's national newsletter. But she never told the doctor; she just left the practice.

You May Not Recognize Jargon, But Patients Do. It's easy to inadvertently use medical terms since this language is so commonly used among all health care professionals. Often what you think of as a commonly understood word or phrase is quite foreign to the patient. Even relatively simple medical terms are widely misinterpreted by patients. Half the people interviewed in a Yale University study thought that *hypertension* meant nervous or easily upset. The patient is "hyper" and "tense." Pediatrician Korsch reported that patients thought lumbar punctures were to drain the lungs, meningitis was a problem in the throat, and the incubation period was thought to mean how long you have to stay in bed (Korsch, Gozzi, and Francis, 1968). Other problem words we have encountered in our workshops include *orally, acute, chronic, fissure, traumatic, anterior, posterior,* and *occlusion.*

Patients' Jargon. Sometimes it's the clinician who struggles to understand the patient's terminology for medical problems. Over the years, clinicians in our workshops have told us of patients who reported such puzzling maladies as this classic: "I got fireballs in the Eucharist and very close veins in my legs, but I'm better off than my sister, who had Final

Mighty Jesus." You may have to struggle awhile to understand this kind of misinterpretation of medical terms—in this case, fibroids, uterus, varicose veins, and spinal meningitis—but even more important here is not to laugh when you finally get it! It's still a condition that concerns the patient, who deserves your professional respect.

One of our physician-participants told us of a frail, elderly woman who resisted for several weeks all attempts to admit her to the hospital for her serious heart problems. Finally the woman confessed in tears that she'd worked as a housecleaner for fifty-five years and was just too weak to be able to do cleaning work anymore. "Who said anything about work?" the cardiologist asked. A nurse had told her that they wanted her in the hospital for "work-up on the seventh floor."

Written and Spoken Jargon Are Not the Same. Some words are understandable when written down but don't translate well into speech. *Asymmetrical, acute,* and *asymptomatic* are examples. Even if the patient understands the written word, when you say, "Right now you seem to be asymptomatic," the patient may answer, "A symptomatic what?" (and "While you're acute . . ." "So you think I'm cute?"). A "fissure" conjures up a picture of someone with a rod and reel, and "traumatic" sounds like a theatrical event on a stage.

Favoring simple language lessens the possibility of patients' consenting to a procedure without fully understanding the risks. It's also a way of letting them know you care enough to explain things in a way they will understand. Here is a list of simple words you can use in place of jargon:

Medical Term	Preferred Term
Obstruction	Blockage
Occlusion	Blockage
Hypertension	High blood pressure
Anterior	Front
Posterior	Back
Trauma	Injury, wound, damage

Contraindicated	Not advisable, to be avoided
Acute	Comes on suddenly, often severely, for a short duration
Chronic	Continuing or lasting a long time, with or without symptoms
Edema	Swelling caused by fluid in the body tissues, as in joints
Metastasize	Spread
Asymptomatic	Having no symptoms
Morbidity	Frequency of the disease
Presents with	Shows symptoms of

Exercise to Remove Communication Barriers

How could you rephrase these explanations to make them more understandable?

1. When coronary angiography reveals severe obstruction in the coronary arteries, then coronary bypass grafting or percutaneous transluminal coronary angioplasty may be indicated.

2. The malignant prostate is generally asymptomatic whereas the benign prostate invariably presents with symptoms, and therefore a comprehensive, annual urological evaluation is indicated.

3. At this point in time, within the medical community it is generally agreed that the oncogene stimulates, in some fashion, the proliferation of malignant cells.

4. In patients who have obstructions in the blood vessels, and who have significant chest pain despite judicious medical management, coronary angiograms are indicated to define their coronary anatomy.

5. Intubation is clearly indicated as the management procedure of choice in such acute situations.

6. It is currently thought that a certain percentile of patients may have a genetic predisposition to malignant hypothermia, which could result in negative patient care outcome.

As an example of simplifying, let's translate just the first item. It could be rephrased as, "When special x-rays of the heart show that the main blood vessels to the heart are clogged, then those blood vessels need to be unclogged, or else they need to be rerouted. If we take the first approach and unblock the vessels, that's called angioplasty. If we take the second method, we reroute the vessels, which is called a coronary bypass. Both approaches have a similar goal: to help your blood flow more easily, more freely, into your heart."

An even simpler approach is, "When we determine through tests that the blood vessels feeding the heart are blocked, they need to be cleaned out or else detoured."

Offer Road Maps

Written instructions or maps given to patients before they leave can be helpful and save time and frustration for you and your patients. Remembering where and when they go for a referral or a test, what to do next after that test or referral appointment, and other important details can be difficult, especially if patients are worried and in a strange environment. A map with arrows or notes directing a patient where to go after the lab work, for example, can eliminate phone calls or returning to ask the receptionist, the busy nurse, or you for instructions.

In a large clinic or hospital setting, patients are often confused about how to find their way around. A small printed map of the clinic, x-ray areas, lab test areas, and the like can help orient the patient. Such maps, similar to those used by concierges at hotels, can be printed on a small pad of customized paper and ripped off, marked with the route, and handed to the patient. Many large clinics and hospitals are already using them. As you write, verbalize the instructions for the patient to hear: "Here's where you are now, here's where you have to go to x-ray, and then here's the lab where you go for your blood work...."

Avoid Alarm Words

Alarm words can terrify patients. For example, at the beginning of this chapter, we saw a cardiologist explain what an angiogram entailed: "We just force a tube into your heart, shoot you with radioactive dye, and light up your vessels." Count the "alarm words" in that one: "force a tube," "shoot," "radioactive," "dye" (doubly dangerous because of its homonym *die*), and "light up the vessels." (As in *my* vessels?) And how about that phrase, "Just force a tube into the heart"? The word *just* is not the appropriate qualifier—ever—for the phrase "force a tube into your heart." We wonder if the doctor would be so nonchalant if he were the patient. A favorite cartoon used in our workshops shows a patient responding to a surgeon: "Oh, I get it. If it's surgery on me, it's minor. If it's surgery on you, it's major!"

Other alarm words or phrases are *rip, force, burn, tear tissue, cut into you,* and *deadly.* Whenever you can find other words that carry less of an emotional load, without losing the meaning you are trying to convey, it's easier on the patient. Patients are already emotionally taut because of their illness, and if they face any surgery or other invasive procedures it compounds their fear. Why add even more stress through something as controllable as your choice of words?

In particular, it's important to avoid clusters of alarm words. In the heart example, using *radioactive* alone might not be a problem, but the doctor uses a cluster of five frightening terms. It's overload for a nervous patient, and the doctor's words can burn some terrifying mental images into the patient's mind.

Avoid "Hot Buttons"

Hot buttons are phrases that we often hear used in clinics and hospitals nationwide. Unlike alarm words, which can frighten patients, hot buttons draw an angry response. They are not patient-friendly and can be infuriating. When you press these hot buttons, patients are diverted from focusing on the information given to them. Although they may not confront you or your staff member at the moment, patients do tend to remember these rude, patronizing phrases, and many even leave a practice because of them. Actually, the patients probably leave because of the underlying attitudes of the health care professional that produce these hot-button comments in the first place. As we mentioned in Chapter Two, patients are guided by their gut-level, intuitive sense of where they get the best care for themselves and their family over the long term.

Here is a sampling of commonly used hot buttons:

Hot Buttons	Substitutes
You'll have to wait . . .	We'll be happy to get that for you as soon as . . .
Now, just calm down.	I can see this is uncomfortable for you. Let's take a while and talk about it.
Now, just take a deep breath.	It seems you're really worried about something. Tell me what worries you. What's your main concern about this?
You have to realize that . . .	The situation is that . . . What we're dealing with here is . . .
You don't understand.	Let's go over that again.
We've already been over that.	I'll say it another way.
OK, I'll go through it—again!	Sure! I want to be certain my explanation is clear.
No, we can't do that.	The situation we're dealing with here is . . . and that's against our policy. What we can do is . . .
I don't have time today.	At our next visit . . .
Not today. I'm running behind.	I want to watch that and follow up on it at our next visit.
(on an answering machine)	
If you *really need* to call me this weekend, I'll be at area code 942 . . .	(Well, what can we say?)

Use a Positive Spin

It is often just as easy to phrase what you say in a positive vein as in the negative, without changing the meaning. Here are some examples.

Negative	Positive
Before we can do this, we'll need . . .	So that we can do that, we need . . . In order to do that, we first need . . .
Your test results won't be back until . . .	Your test results should be back within (state a range of time that is realistic, such as "a week or two").

Here are a few others. See how quickly you can give them a quick spin in the positive direction.

Negative	Positive
I can't think of any reason not to. I don't have any objections. I don't like to say no, but . . . If nothing goes wrong, you should be able to . . .	

A veteran internist who has had a successful practice for many years told us: "I never say to a patient, 'You may have to live with that pain the rest of your life.' Instead I tell my patients that no matter what the situation, even if it's a chronic condition, I will do my very best to help them—however I can. It's the glass half-full rather than half-empty."

"But" Out

Try using the word *and* in place of the word *but*. You may be surprised how often you can do that without significantly changing the meaning of your sentence.

Negative: "Ms. Sullivan, I see you're due for a tetanus shot, but we can't do that until you bring in your vaccination records."

Positive: "Ms. Sullivan, I see you're due for a tetanus shot, and we'll be happy to do that for you when you bring in your vaccination records."

Negative: "You'll need to have an x-ray, but that department is closed now."

Positive: "You'll need to have an x-ray, and although that department is closed now, you can have your x-rays done between eight in the morning and five in the afternoon any day this week."

"Up" Ended

End your explanation on a positive, upbeat note whenever possible. This can be what you hope will happen, or it can be the benefit you hope to gain from the treatment plan you've just outlined. If you try, you can probably find something positive or encouraging to say without getting into false-hope issues: "Let's see how we do with this new program, Mrs. Levine. You said you'd like to lose some pounds to feel better and have more pep. Let's hope this new plan will help you reach your goal. Next month, when you go to visit those grandchildren, it would be nice to have plenty of energy to keep up with them!"

Elicit the Patient's Service Expectation

After you explain what you think is the best treatment approach for a patient, it is also important to get feedback. It may not be at all what that patient wanted or is hoping for. As we pointed out in Chapter Three, some patients, especially those of the Amiable social style, may not tell you if they are displeased with your methods or if they don't understand why you are choosing that particular approach. Questions to elicit the patient's reaction include "How do you feel about that?" or "What are your thoughts on this approach?"

Prompting in this way to get the patient's reaction is often left out by busy clinicians who have other patients waiting. We recommend it, however, because by catching any dissatisfaction before the patient leaves, you can affect the patient's adherence to the therapies you've prescribed. In addition, if the patient is really unhappy about something, it may be the last time you see that patient.

Here are other phrases you can use to determine the patient's expectation of service:

- "How do you feel about that?"
- "Are you comfortable with this plan?"
- "Does this seem reasonable?"
- "What are your thoughts on that?"
- "When you came in today, you probably had some ideas of how I could help you. . . ."
- "What were you hoping I could do for you today?"
- "I like to encourage my patients to share their thoughts with me so I know whether we're on track. What were you expecting or hoping we might do for you today?"

Occasional checks such as these, to see that you and the patient are congruent in your goals and your expectations, can insure against a sudden, unexpected glitch in your communications regarding care.

Giving explanations to patients consumes a large portion of your day. We hope the tips and suggestions in this chapter help you conserve time and get the most value for you and your patients from the minutes you have with them. In addition, we believe these suggestions can reduce the problems that arise from misunderstanding of your explanations.

But there are other, more important goals in these communication techniques: (1) to increase the probability that patients will adhere more faithfully to your recommendations because they understand them and remember them, (2) that your patients will be more motivated and committed to their treatment plans because of the way you involve them in the explanation and discussion, and (3) that patients will be comforted by the caring manner in which you convey your medical knowledge—a manner that helps them through their fears and pain.

CHAPTER 7

Communicating About Medications

The thirty-four-year-old construction worker and his wife are being seen in the exam room. He does most of the talking and decision making for his shy wife. Confused and perturbed, he says that on their last visit two years ago, the doctor wrote a prescription for birth control pills and that he immediately saw to having it filled. Since then, he complains, his wife has given birth to an infant and is now pregnant again. There are five other children at home.

"Why?" he asks the doctor. "Why don't the pills work?" The physician probes: "Is it the right pill?" It is. "Is the pill being taken on schedule?" Absolutely! The man pulls a small calendar from his workman's shirt pocket to show the days checked off. Every day, right on schedule, he takes the pill.

It may seem preposterous, but we have heard this scenario and similar stories of misunderstood instructions many times from participants in our workshops, both physicians and other health care professionals.

If there is one thing that absolutely must be accomplished during your patient's visit, it's making sure you've communicated to the patient an essential understanding of his or her treatment regimen. Every day, one out of three patients walks out of the doctor's office without being given any information on how often to take the medications or how much is to be taken, according to national surveys by the Food and Drug Administration (1998).

Medications are prescribed in about three-fifths (63 percent) of all medical visits in the United States (National Center for Health Statistics, 1999). That's a lot of potential for mistakes. And the potential is often realized—unfortunately. According to many researchers (including DiMatteo, 1994), up to half the medications prescribed by physicians and other health care professionals are not taken correctly by their patients.

This chapter offers suggestions and techniques—to add to those you already use—for explaining clearly how to take medications and for checking to make sure your patients understand their medications.

You may ask, "If patients are walking out of their doctors' offices without all their questions answered, why don't they just speak up and ask their doctors how to take the medications correctly?" There are many reasons they don't. One is the difference in perceived status between the physician and patient, which often causes timidity and passivity in patients. Only 1 percent of patients asked their doctors how much medication to take or how often to take it, according to the FDA National Consumer Survey (Food and Drug Admnistration, 1998). Whatever the reason patients don't speak up and ask these important questions, it's clear that, like the worker and his pregnant wife at the beginning of this chapter, many just don't.

Because patients don't ask, doctors can easily take a no-news-is-good-news attitude and assume patients don't have any questions. This dangerous spiral of patients who don't question and clinicians who don't explain can be slowed by new awareness of the need for a more collaborative and less authoritarian style of interaction between clinicians and patients. Patients themselves are becoming more proactive about their health care, fortified by frequent reminders in the national media about the importance of asking questions and taking an assertive role in their own care.

But the situation of patients improperly taking medications or stopping them still persists, and whatever the reasons for this breakdown in communication, the clinician's exam room or office is where the main repair work needs to begin. Only 35 percent of patients were told by their physicians how often to take their medications, according to a recent FDA survey (Food and Drug Administration, 1998), and only 32 percent were told how much to take. Sixty-three percent were not told of any precautions at all about taking their medications. It remains your responsibility to make sure your patients understand how, when, and for how long to take their medications and that you sufficiently motivate them, before they leave your office, to stick to the regimen.

Taking medications incorrectly contributes to prolonged illnesses, avoidable side effects, life-threatening interactions, unnecessary hospitalizations, and, of course, even deaths.

ESSENTIAL INFORMATION ABOUT MEDICATION

Before your patients leave your office, clinic, or hospital, there is essential information they must have. Here are the basics your patients need to know about their medications, especially new prescriptions, as recommended by the National Council on Patient Information and Education (2000):

- What is the name of the medicine, and what is it supposed to do? Is this the brand or generic name?
- How and when does the patient take the medicine, and for how long?
- What foods, drinks, or other medicines or activities should be avoided while taking it?
- What are the possible side effects, and what should the patient do if they occur?
- Will this new prescription work safely with other prescription and nonprescription medicines or with any dietary supplements the patient may be taking?
- Why is it important to take the medication according to instructions?
- Is any written information about the medication available? Any in large print or in the patient's native tongue, if either is necessary?
- Should the medicine be refilled? If so, when?
- How should the medicine be stored?
- When should the medication begin to work, and how will the patient know it is working?

Here are some useful tips for increasing the likelihood that patients will understand and adhere to their prescribed medications.

GENERAL TECHNIQUES TO ENHANCE YOUR EXPLANATIONS ABOUT MEDICATIONS

Holding a patient's attention requires staying tuned in to that person's interests and level of comprehension. Following are a number of ways to get your important messages across.

Go to the Patient's Starting Point First

Before you launch into an explanation about a medication, it's important to know the patient's starting point first. This includes what the patient already knows about the medication or the treatment plan, as well as what attitudes, experiences, and beliefs the patient has about the particular medication or class of medications A simple question or two—"Have you ever taken this medication?" and then, "What was your experience with it?"—can establish the patient's level of understanding.

Personalize the Body Parts in Your Explanation

Instead of saying "the shoulder" or "the lungs," try saying "your shoulder," "your blood vessels," "your joints," and so forth. It may not always be appropriate to do so, but use the personal *you* or *your* whenever possible. This recognizes the patient as a unique individual, rather than as a clinically interesting textbook phenomenon. It's easy to do and takes no additional time to phrase your explanation in this personally interested way. In addition, when you talk about "your vessels," the patient is more likely to feel the impact of the message and be more motivated to follow the regimen. It's subtle but effective and sends the message, "This is your body we're talking about, not some remote medical case study."

Monitor your own pattern of speaking, and see how often you say "the blood vessels," "the heart," "the headaches," and so forth, when you could say "your blood vessels," "your heart," and the like.

Avoid Information Overload

You probably tell twenty or thirty people a week how to take antibiotics and what to watch for, or how to use an inhaler properly, but it may be the first time your patient has heard it.

If you say, "Furosemide, or Lasix, is a diuretic that dilates your vessels and reduces heart rate, thereby alleviating congestive symptoms," you may be giving the patient too much information in terms too clinical to assimilate. Unfamiliar with these terms and emotionally tense, the patient may just shut down and stop listening.

Give One Key Point per Sentence

We suggest that if the information is important, new, and somewhat complex, try giving the patient only one big dose of medical data to swallow per sentence. This will help to avoid possible information overload. Here is an example of how you can explain and educate at the same time. Notice there is one concept or medical term per sentence:

- There is a class of drugs known as diuretics, or water pills.
- Diuretics help your kidneys to get rid of extra fluids in your body.
- The particular form of diuretic that I am recommending for you is a medication called Lasix.
- Lasix, being one of these diuretics, can help your body rid itself of extra water.
- Getting rid of the extra water in your body is important because it means your heart doesn't have to work so hard to circulate (or pump around) the fluids in your system.
- When your heart doesn't have to work so hard—because it has less fluid to pump—you will probably feel better and have fewer symptoms.

You might want to add:

Lasix is also known as a furosemide, which is its generic name. But usually when you and I talk about this medication, we'll call it Lasix.

Use Pauses

Use pauses to let the information sink in—to let patients consider how they will incorporate this new situation into their daily lives. As with the natural pause in your voice that a period at the end of a sentence usually engenders, you can also separate complex concepts and essential information by simply pausing two beats between these units of information as you speak.

Let's say that this is what you normally tell a patient:

> You will need to take this antibiotic, called _____, three times a day with meals and continue to take the pills for ten days, until all the pills are gone. Be sure to take this medication with food so it's easier on your stomach, and it's also important to drink lots of fluids, about six to eight glasses a day, and get plenty of rest. I'd like to see you back in about two weeks.

It is easier for many patients to assimilate all this if you build in pauses of a few beats—about two seconds—between units of important information. It allows the patient a mental breather to catch up and to assimilate the flow of data coming from you. Here's an example:

> You will need to take this antibiotic, . . . which is called _____, three times a day . . . and be sure you take it with meals. . . . Continue to take the pills for about ten days . . . or until all the pills in the container are gone. . . . If you take this medication with food, . . . it will be easier on your stomach.

As you do this, be sure to use the techniques for simple, jargon-free explanations that we described earlier in this chapter—for example, "Atenolol is a medication that helps to slow down your heart rate. It opens your blood vessels wider so that the blood can flow more easily through them."

TECHNIQUES FOR AVOIDING MEDICATION DROPOUTS

You're better off preparing ahead for those moments when patients are likely to be most vulnerable to not following their medication regimen. Here are some ways to do that.

Anticipate and Address Hurdles with the Patient

Those "Who needs this!" moments will come, as statistics clearly indicate, with at least one of every two patients not fully following their doctors' recommendations on their prescribed drugs (Roter and Hall, 1992). It's better that you both discuss and deal with the possible dropout points while the patient is still with you, rather than having to deal with the person in the middle of the night when there could be a serious problem resulting from the patient's not taking the medication correctly.

Questions that are helpful in determining when the patient is most likely to waver from the treatment plan include:

• What difficulties, if any, do you think you might have in filling this prescription and taking this medication on schedule?

• How will this fit into your day?

• What adjustments will you need to make so you can take the medications at the times we discussed? What do you think might help?

• Since you indicated that it will be difficult for you to take this three times a day, how would taking a once-a-day form of this medication work for you?

• What problems do you see arising that might possibly interfere with your continuing this medication?

Most of the questions we suggest for discussing possible hurdles are open-ended, to encourage your patients to tell you about their situation or their attitudes toward taking a medication as prescribed.

Ask the Tough Questions Gingerly and Privately

Some questions have a significant emotional charge attached, perhaps conjuring up a sense of embarrassment or shame in the patient. You will have to prompt the patient gently to open up about these. "Tell me more about the stomach problems you had with the previous antibiotics." "You mentioned some problems in terms of your sexual relations with your wife since you started on the medications. How would you describe those problems?" "You mentioned feeling a little down lately; let's talk more about that."

Circle Around and Come Back Later

If you ask one of these difficult questions—even after you've established a good relationship, using the listening techniques we recommend—but you still don't get an answer, or you suspect it's not a complete answer, you can do what many investigative journalists do. They leave that topic for a while and come back from a different direction later and ask it again, rephrased so it's not likely to be recognized as a repeated question. Try to stay with an open-ended question, and be sure you rephrase it on the second asking.

Give Patients Scenarios to Help Them Remember

Another way you can anticipate the points where patients might stop using medications is by warning your patients about your past experience with patients who stopped. Keep it general, of course, with no information that identifies a particular patient. For example:

> Often my patients will feel much better after taking these antibiotics for a few days, and that's when they tend to think—"Oh, I'm better now. I don't really need to keep taking these pills." But even if you're feeling better—and I hope you will be—it's still important to keep on taking all the pills in the bottle. I stress this because if you don't, it's possible the bronchitis could come back. Neither one of us wants that, so be sure to take all the pills in this container until they are completely gone.

Check for Financial Hurdles

I always stop at the on-site pharmacy of health care clients when first arriving to present workshops for them. It is amazing to discover the piles of prescription medications that are never picked up—often because the prescribing clinician didn't realize the patient couldn't pay for the medications.

To anticipate this potential hurdle with patients, you might try a few gentle probes. For many people, pride may not allow a candid answer to a question such as "Can you afford this?" That's why, if you suspect this issue needs to be addressed, it is better to ask about this when you are alone with the patient. Also, be sure to begin with open-ended questions, since they are not as easy to toss off with an "Oh, sure." You have to choose an approach that fits your own style best. Here are a few suggestions to get you started:

- "I realize this is a new addition to your monthly expenses. So I usually check with my patients just to be sure the medications can be purchased today so we can get started right away. But you will be taking this for several months, and maybe longer, so how will this new, added expense work out for you?"
- "We just spoke about some of the hurdles you might face in taking this medication. For many patients, another hurdle is just fitting the cost of the medications into their budget. It can squeeze things a bit." Look at the patient, and wait for a few seconds for a response.
- "In the past, some of my patients have waited to pick up their medications until the end of the month, when their checks come in. Often that's too long to delay starting the medication. So now, I generally double-check with all my patients just to be certain they can pick up the medications right away. If cost is a concern, there may be a generic medication or another less expensive medication that can be prescribed."

If this gentler probing doesn't elicit a clear answer and you suspect the cost of the medication could be an issue, you might need to ask directly, "What about the cost of these medications? Is that a manageable added expense, or does it present difficulties?" Or simply, "Will you be able to afford these medications?"

Let the Patient Know the Dosage May Need Adjusting

Steve, a twenty-nine-year-old stockbroker who is experiencing seizures, is told by the neurologist that the medication she recommends is the best for his situation; she feels quite sure this will bring good results in controlling the problem.

Two weeks later, Steve has several more seizures. "This doctor doesn't know what she's doing! That's it—I'm *done!*" he announces to his family. His father, however, encourages Steve to tell the neurologist what's occurring.

"This is still the best medication for your problem," she says. Steve protests loudly that it sure doesn't seem that way to him—not after a seizure during a business lunch with important clients! "Of course," she replies, "that's because we haven't yet reached the dosage needed to control the seizures. We have to start this medication in smaller doses and gradually work up to the point where the seizures can be controlled."

"Why didn't she tell me that?!" Steve complains to his family later. He was ready to give up on both the medication and the doctor. "She never laid out the plan. She didn't let me know when this stuff kicks in," he fumes, understandably angry that the neurologist didn't take a few moments to explain and to involve him in the process.

When you prescribe a medication that may need to be adjusted, tell the patient. Explain that although you have chosen this medication specifically for your patient's situation, hoping to get the desired results, the fact is, medications react differently in various patients. You both need to watch, see how it works, and stay in contact.

Discuss Possible Side Effects Before They Happen

When you tell the patient up front that the medication may not be immediately effective or may produce unpleasant but often manageable side effects, the patient is less likely to abandon the medication out of frustration if it doesn't produce the desired effect immediately or if there are unpleasant side effects. You are also less likely to be blamed or thought incompetent by the patient. A good approach, which Lanny uses

174

with his patients, is to say, "The medication you're taking is what you need. But if there are side effects, we can alter the dosage to one that works best for you. Our goal is to find a balance between unwanted side effects and the dosage of this medicine that you need to help your blood pressure [or other medical situation]."

Be candid about side effects of medications and clarify, if necessary, with statistics. Physicians in our workshops say that some of the printed materials that patients receive with their medications use potentially frightening phrases that begin, "Some patients experience . . ." and don't cite the actual statistical probabilities involved, which may be as low as 1 or 2 percent.

Dealing with Media Reports

The media can affect how, or if, patients take medications as you prescribed them. If patients read or hear disturbing reports about new studies of a medicine or class of medicines through a news broadcast, this can raise concerns if they are taking those medicines. If you are aware of this kind of recent coverage in the media, you might want to anticipate the patient's concern. Do this while the patient is in your office if possible. "You may see reports about [name of the medication] in the media lately. What we know at this time is . . . [and provide the appropriate explanation]."

Check for "Negative Reactions" to a Medication

Finding out the patient's attitudes and past experiences can profoundly affect adherence and save time and problems later.

Two minutes spent carefully explaining how to use an inhaler to a patient who is secretly terrified of inhalers and absolutely will not use it is two minutes probably wasted.

Telling a patient about forcing fluids and taking aspirin or acetaminophen is lost time if the patient is convinced that antibiotics are really what is needed, leaves your office, goes home, and perhaps takes a relative's leftover antibiotic prescription.

That's why we suggest you elicit the patient's experiences and health beliefs about a medication first before you jump into your own routine explanation of it. We touched on this earlier in this chapter under the heading "Go to the Patient's Starting Point First." If your patient is firmly opposed to taking an antibiotic, your time is better spent by asking about that, using open-ended questions:

- What are your main concerns about taking this medication?

- What do you think might happen if you take this?

- When you came in today, what were you hoping I might do for you instead of prescribing this medication?

First pinpointing and dealing with the patient's attitudes and concerns about the medication is essential, since it can profoundly affect that patient's adherence. Once you know the concerns or negative attitudes, you can adjust the discussion and deal with those first. Otherwise you're probably losing time—and maybe a patient as well.

In the case of a patient with a virus-based URI who insists on an antibiotic, you might choose to explain why antibiotics are not useful in combating a virus. For a patient with arthritis, you might learn that the probability of the patient's taking an NSAID three times a day is very low and that a medication with a once-a-day dosage is a more realistic alternative.

Perhaps a patient was expecting to receive a particular medication but his insurance doesn't cover it, or your pharmacy doesn't carry that one but has another medication with a similar chemical makeup. You need to explain why the medication you are recommending is a good alternative, thereby assuaging his fears or misgivings.

But you can't know which of these paths to take until you first determine the patient's experiences with and attitude toward the medication. Asking a good open-ended question or two can give you that essential information.

Start Patients Off with a Positive Attitude

If you have had good results with other patients using a medication in the past, you might (as part of your explanation) tell your patient that too. They love to hear the success stories of others who have been in their situation. Don't give specific names or identifying information, of course, but just a simple comment: "Several of my patients have had very good results with this medication, and we'll hope that you will too" can help put the patient in an upbeat frame of mind. The patient may have a positive attitude toward the medication right from the start. Say this, however, only if you and your other patients actually have had good results with the medication.

Be Aware of Interactions with Folk or Alternative Remedies

It's impossible to watch TV, ride a bus, or visit a mall without seeing a multitude of advertisements praising the effectiveness of herbs and dietary supplements for treating all sorts of conditions. In addition, many patients grew up in ethnic settings with—and remain loyal to—"folk medicine." The emergence of alternative medicine requires greater caution in advising patients about prescription medicines.

The following types of questions can be especially important if there's any chance the patient may also be using an herbal remedy, such as an herbal tea or other type of alternative therapy that could interact unfavorably with what you are prescribing.

- What other medications have you tried for this in the past?

- What else seems to work when you are sick (*or* when this recurs, etc.)?

- Is there anything else that helps when you have this? How did that seem to work for you?

- What home remedies have you tried?

If patients divulge that they are using a self-selected or home remedy, such as vitamin therapy, do not instantly disparage it with words or with demeaning body language (a shoulder shrug or an exasperated wag of the head). Discuss it openly, with respect and a nonjudgmental attitude toward your patient's views and beliefs. If you don't, it's likely to be the last time you hear about these remedies from that patient.

Conduct Regular Medication Checkups

Go over all the medications the patient is currently taking, over-the-counter as well as prescription. Doing a comprehensive inventory can prevent duplicating medications, as well as uncover situations of overdosing and possible medication buildup, especially in older patients. It allows you to double-check that there are no undesirable interactions among medications being taken concurrently. It is best if you have patients bring all their medications in to you (probably in the proverbial brown bag) so you can see what the medications and dosages are and how the patient is taking them, as well as check expiration dates. If there are too many pills left in a bottle and they should have been finished, for example, you have an important warning about that patient's probable lack of adherence.

Reviewing all medications for a particular patient affords another good opportunity to ask about side effects: "How are you doing with this medication?" Then wait for the answer; if none comes, use the closed-ended, direct version: "Have you noticed any side effects?"

Whether it's at medication reviews, regular patient follow-up appointments, or any future medical visits, check with patients to see how the medications they are taking are working for them; check the dosage and also ask about the status of any new medications they may now be taking. As you do so, try to keep your questions open-ended. We mention in Chapter Five that this approach opens up patient secrets. Closed-ended questions are too easy to wiggle out of answering ("Any problems with the new medications?" "No." "Any difficulty sleeping at night?" "No." "Feeling OK?" "Sure.").

Make It Easy to Take Medications

Many patients who have diseases such as severe arthritis find prescription vials difficult to open. You could arrange for a container cap that is easier to twist off than the childproof variety. Or the patient can put rubber bands around the neck of the container to get a better grip while opening it. Colored rubber bands, available in many variety stores, allow for color-coding the prescription vials at the same time. Older patients often have difficulty seeing which medication they are taking. A colored marker drawn over the top of the medication container is another way to color-code and can help prevent taking the wrong medications.

For patients who have poor eyesight, bits of sandpaper or Velcro dots stuck on the top of a container are a tactile cue as to which medication is which.

You may prefer to have someone on your staff explain to your patients about these various aids to making it easier for them to take medications.

TIPS TO HELP YOU REMEMBER THE ESSENTIAL POINTS

The results and the benefits you and your patients realize from using any medication can be significantly affected by how well they understand the essential information and comply with your instructions. But how can you be sure you remember to tell them all these essentials?

Give Patients the Full Story

One technique to be sure you've covered the critical information is to go down the list of open-ended question starters: *who, what, when, where, why, how,* and *how much.* These are also the key words reporters use to be sure they've covered all the essential points in a news story. You may re-member these from your own classes in English.

Who Questions. A *who* question focuses on the patient, since that is whom you have selected this particular medication for. Tell the patient why you have selected it specifically for him or her, at this time, given the specific situation. This is another opportunity for a benefits message. One of the reasons the patient comes to you is to have your expertise and rec-ommendation regarding appropriate ways to help what hurts or is of con-cern. So explain why you think this is in your patient's best interest and what results you are hoping for. You can do this without raising any false hopes by adding a phrase such as "We'll hope this gives us the results we both want for you."

Another *who* issue is that the patient should not take the medicine of another "who"—such as a family member or friend who has taken this drug and may have leftover supplies. In fact, 12–20 percent of patients take other people's medicines (Young, 1987). According to many of the participants in our workshops, there is much "over-the-fence" medication sharing as well as use of medications purchased at swap meets, often with expired dates.

What Questions. *What* questions include "What is the name of the drug?" "What is it supposed to do?" "What should you watch for?" and "What should you avoid while taking it—food or activities, for example?"

In answer to the first one, give not only the generic name and the product name but the category, too: "This is a medication that is part of a larger group known as 'beta blockers.'" If the patient has a chronic disease and is to take this medication for a long period of time, it is especially important to educate him in this way, giving the name and category of medicine.

Describing what the medication is supposed to do is important because this is what may keep the patient motivated to follow the regimen. In addition, your explanation tends to make the patient feel a partnership with you.

The response to "What should you watch for?" addresses possible side effects. Many health care professionals don't like to tell their patients about side effects out of concern that patients will then have imaginary symptoms. But we recommend you tell patients the major ones at least so that they can be watchful. They are likely to be more disappointed if they have side effects and were not told about them. "What to watch for" also includes indicators that a medication is working.

When Questions. *When* questions are those that concern the actual schedule for the medication. When is this drug to be taken? Three times a day?

Two pills first thing in the morning? If an antibiotic is prescribed to be taken every eight hours, does the parent have to awaken the child in the middle of the night, or can it be given three times during daytime hours? If the medication is to be taken with meals, this may pose problems for a shift worker who doesn't have "regular" meals, or who has breakfast at 3:00 A.M.

If a medication is to be taken three times a day, get the patient's input as to what are convenient and easily remembered times during the day to take the medication. To answer, the patient has to give it some thought and see himself taking the medication at particular times of the day: "Since you will be taking this medication three times a day, what would be easier to remember: if you took it at breakfast, lunch, and dinner, or at bedtime instead of at dinner?" This conjures up visual images in the patient's mind of having a meal or going to bed. Seeing a picture or visual image of taking the medication reinforces the verbal explanation and increases the likelihood that the patient will remember.

Another advantage of letting patients have some say in determining aspects of how to fit their medications into their day is that when they are actively involved in the medication planning, even on small issues like exact hours or events connected with dosage, they are likely to adhere to the plan, since they helped design it.

Where Questions. *Where* questions get down to the issue of logistics. Where will patients be when they take their medicine? Eating a meal? At work or school? Catching a plane for a business trip, which means she could easily miss a dose? Will the patient be leaving on vacation, which may mean taking a copy of the prescription for refills should the medication be lost or forgotten?

Why Questions. Properly asked, *why* questions enhance the patient's understanding that it is essential to take the medication, and to take it according to your instructions. Patients need to have clearly in mind the why of this prescription. Since there will come a point, sometime after leaving your office, when the patient will most likely waver, this can be important information to give all patients, particularly if there may be undesirable side effects, which you will need to know about so you can adjust the dosage of the medication.

What Clinicians Leave Out Most Often

As a regular feature of our workshop role plays, a clinician takes the role of a patient who has been diagnosed with high blood pressure. Another workshop participant plays the prescribing clinician and gives an explanation about the medication. Throughout the fifteen years that Desmond Medical Communications has been presenting workshops, it has been quite surprising to us that only three clinicians out of the hundreds playing this prescribing role have told the patient what could happen if they stop taking their blood pressure medication. Why is such important information not given to the patient, particularly when we know, from many sources, that half the patients to whom you give any medication will probably not take it as you recommend, and may even drop it entirely?

Perhaps telling patients the potential consequences of terminating their medication is not mentioned because of the legacy of the old biomedical approach to explanations, which tends to use a "tell only" approach and invites little or no feedback from the patient. This type of traditional, authoritarian communication carries the assumption that the patient will listen and then go out and do exactly what the doctor said.

We know now that this is simply not a valid assumption. We need to reexamine explanations about medicine to include this important piece of information—in an appropriate manner. It may not be necessary for absolutely all patients but it certainly should be part of the explanation if the consequences of not taking the medication correctly or stopping it could be serious. For example, you might say, "If you should decide not to continue taking the medications, there could be serious consequences, such as . . ."

How Questions (How, How Much, and How Long). A *how* question refers to how this medication is taken. Is it taken by mouth? Is it a suppository? Big difference! We've heard lots of reports from clinicians—and so have you, probably—about these getting mixed up.

A *how much* question tells how much of the medication is to be taken. A patient may want to know if a teaspoon is the same as the spoon you stir your tea with.

A *how long* question tells the period of time the medication is to be taken. When can the medication be stopped? Is this a long-term medication to be continued until otherwise instructed? I have also been surprised to see in workshop role plays that when a medication may need to be taken long term, such as a blood pressure medication, the patient is quite often not told that.

Over-the-Counter Medications

If you are suggesting an over-the-counter medication, it will probably have more impact on the patient if you write down the name of the medication and the recommended strength. Writing the name of the medication on a notepad with your name imprinted at the top is more effective and looks more serious than if you say, "Just go to the pharmacy and pick up some Dimetapp." Patients are likely to take it seriously and follow your instructions.

MAKING SURE PATIENTS UNDERSTAND

Once you've given a number of instructions, you'll want to make sure the patient understands what you have said. Here are a few techniques to help you verify that your patient is clear as to the treatment regimen.

Write It Down

Since Desmond Medical Communications surveys indicate that clinicians attribute 21 percent of patients' poor listening to their vagueness and disorientation, this certainly points up the need to write down the information for any patients who seem vague or disoriented, at the very least. But the fact is, if they are nervous or concerned about their health, people of all ages and backgrounds have trouble remembering.

Over the years, I have asked the clinicians in our workshops how many of them actually write down instructions for their patients. Only about one out of four say they do, and many tell me they write instructions down only for their elderly patients because "they might have trouble remembering."

We suggest writing down important instructions for all patients—at least the key points that are important to remember. Research tells us that the patient forgets about one-half of the clinician's statements almost immediately (Ley, Bradshaw, and Eaves, 1973). This is why we think it's important to write down the essential instructions. Also give patients educational pamphlets, drawings, or anything else they can see or read to reinforce the information.

If patients have the information clearly written down, they are more likely to adhere to the treatment plan. The probability of their forgetting, misinterpreting, calling back, or coming back is also lessened—so it clearly pays to take a moment and jot down the essential information you want them to remember and act on.

You may need to work on improving your handwriting, or revert to printing the information. Or, as pharmacies do for medications, you can provide instructions that have been preprinted, perhaps using a word processor. These handouts can then be customized by you or your staff as needed. Again, we suggest that you write the patient's name by hand on the materials. Check off a few places they need to read in particular, which further personalizes the handout.

Writing down the key points can be done without taking additional time if you combine it with your final summing up at the end of the visit. As you verbalize, write down the key points you want the patient to remember when she gets home. It tends to be harder for any of us to focus on facts and data when we are fearful and concerned. As Billings and

Communicating with Today's Patient

Stoeckle point out, "What brings a patient in to see you is an emotion—typically a concern about their health status" (1989, p. 103).

Verify That the Patient Understands

Summaries of important information at the end of the visit can help to drive home whatever point is most important. But these summaries work best if the patient is involved in them; it is most effective if the patient is the one giving the summary. When we ask physicians in our workshop how they check to make sure the patient understands the instructions, the response is usually, "Well, I ask the patient to repeat it back to me" or, in the case of medications, "I say, 'Now, tell me how you'll be taking the medications.'" Some patients resent this approach. They feel put on the spot; "Now, tell me back what I told you" sets up a parent-child or teacher-student dynamic.

But the fact remains, you do need to know if the patient understands. We recommend another approach that is more patient-friendly and less intimidating for them. Instead of putting the responsibility on the patient, you take the responsibility for needing the explanation. For example, you might say, "We've covered a lot here. Just so I'm sure I was clear in my explanation, let's go over how you'll be taking these medications." Or, "Just so I'm sure we covered all the main points, let's review together when you take this."

A recent study of the closing portion of medical visits showed that physicians checked for patient understanding in only 34 percent of the interactions observed. Patients were asked whether they had any more questions in only one out of every four interactions (White, Levinson, and Roter, 1994).

Check for Other Questions

One way to do this allows the patient to "help": "It would help me to know what other questions you might have about this." Or you could ask straightforwardly, "What other questions do you have about this medication and how you'll be taking it?" This is better than asking, "Do you have any questions about this?" Such a closed-ended question, particularly if said in a clipped tone, carries a high risk of getting an inaccurate answer.

Checking Can Save You Time

Many clinicians hesitate to prompt for questions, fearing it might open up another ten minutes of questions—all requiring answers. But it is more efficient to deal with these issues while the patient is sitting in front of you rather than sometime later, perhaps in the middle of the night on the telephone—or in the emergency room.

These tips and techniques for discussing medications with your patients can increase the likelihood that patients will adhere to their medications, resulting in optimum benefits and improved outcomes.

Family members can also play an important role in helping their loved ones adhere to their medications, as well as providing other important assistance to your patient. We offer some essential pointers for communicating with family members in the next chapter.

CHAPTER 8

Effectively Interacting with the Patient's Family

What conditions make it difficult to deal with patients? Approximately 600 physicians and other clinicians who attended Desmond Medical Communications workshops over a six-year period were asked that question. Among the top three most frequent responses was, "They are accompanied by relatives who are difficult to deal with."

It seems that difficulty dealing with relatives is more of a problem than difficulty dealing with patients, in many cases. For example, patients who consistently ramble on about topics unrelated to their medical visit, or those who come in with long lists of physical complaints, don't present as much of a challenge as insistent or angry relatives, according to this survey. The only categories of difficult encounters that rated higher were angry, hostile patients, an understandable first choice, and patients who appear to be trying to manipulate the clinician to get what they want.

We used a multiple-choice questionnaire, circulated to primary care physicians, physician assistants, and nurse practitioners associated with nine health care organizations in five states. The survey, which covered a six-year period, was statistically analyzed by Margaret H. DeFleur, Ph.D., director of the graduate program in health communication at Boston University's College of Communication (DeFleur and Desmond, forthcoming). Dealing with demanding and complaining family members was also cited as a problem in another study of physician frustration in communicating with patients (Levinson, Stiles, Inui, and Engle, 1993).

These combined findings make it imperative, we believe, to devote one chapter to specifically addressing techniques for communicating with family members. Keeping the relationship with family members on a positive track can reduce tensions and make your work easier, often creating three-way synergy to support you, the patient, and the family members.

THE PATIENT'S CHAMPION

Why do clinicians find patients' relatives so difficult to deal with? Anyone who has ever taken a sick child or elderly parent to the hospital or to a doctor's appointment is probably aware of being far more assertive on behalf of the loved one than he would ever be for himself.

Sometimes the family members are adult children of an older patient, in reverse parent-child roles. They often feel responsible for their vulnerable loved one—perhaps with an accompanying sense of wanting to pay back the parent for the years of loving care they received as children.

Clinicians in our workshops have also described other situations in which adult children who have not visited their elderly parents for a considerable length of time nonetheless fly quickly to the hospital bedside and vigorously demonstrate to Mom or Dad how much they care and how active they will be on their parent's behalf. Some clinicians observe dryly that perhaps this helps assuage guilt for long periods of neglect. Whatever the reason, health care professionals may be caught in the middle.

A more common scenario, however, is that family members are just frustrated and angry that they can't get information about the patient to ease their concerns. This is important information that is likely to have a profound impact on their lives and on their loved one. This may well be a major passage to them—a turning point—in their lives, even though to you it's another day in your professional life. A casual "we'll let you know when it's convenient" attitude can suddenly ignite the frazzled nerves of these distraught family members, causing an explosion of pent-up emotions.

GENERAL TIPS FOR COMMUNICATING
WITH FAMILY MEMBERS

There are ways to manage this type of situation, however. Here are some communication tips and techniques for communicating successfully with family members. Adjust them to your own style and take as needed.

Make Them Your Allies

Reframe the whole portrait of family members. Rather than seeing them as potential problem makers, which many clinicians do (particularly after one or two unpleasant run-ins), keep in mind that they can be important cohorts in successfully managing your patient's illness. Family members or special friends who come with the patient can be your valuable supporters, often acting as dedicated, unpaid home health aides.

Enlist the Support of Family Members

If your patient agrees, include family members, particularly a spouse or other life partner, in your interactions with the patient. The modifications in lifestyle that are frequently required with chronic illnesses in particular—changes in diet or physical activity—often affect the entire family. Clinical trials have shown that significant improvement in how faithfully patients keep appointments, take their medications as they were prescribed, and stick to the treatment plan can be realized when a member of the family is involved in the treatment (Levine, 1989).

Comfort Your Patient by Relating with Family

Since friends and family members are the patient's main support system, both physically and emotionally, it can be very comforting to the patient to know that you communicate in a respectful and considerate way with them. One of the seven essential "Dimensions of Care" identified by Dr. Thomas Delbanco and colleagues through research and focus groups with patients includes the patient's interest in involving family and friends, particularly in terms of planning and providing ongoing care (Delbanco, 1992).

Take a Moment to Focus on Them Right at the Start

A few moments to show your interest in and your respect for the patient's family members at the beginning of the visit is courteous and helps to get the relationship off to a good start. Ask their names and their relationship to the patient. Use good body language as you do this, or you will lose the value of the time spent. Be sure your shoulders are oriented toward them as you meet and greet each person in the family. Have good eye contact and, if appropriate, a smile. Keep your movements somewhat slow and gracious at this point to show that establishing a relationship with them is important and that you are not just bolting through this as a perfunctory task before rushing on to the next problem.

Each time these family members come back in future visits, take a moment to greet them, preferably using their names. This courteous welcome goes a long way in showing your respect and in maintaining their positive perception of you.

Give Family Members a Task

There are a variety of helpful tasks the patient's family members can do, including shopping for or preparing special foods, recording medications or overseeing a physical therapy regimen, and keeping track of liquids consumed. Ask the family members first, of course, if they are willing and can conveniently perform some of these simple but helpful tasks. These contributions should be truly helpful and not just make-work for family members. And clearly, the task must not be something that only a skilled health care professional should be doing.

If the family member is given a helpful task, she is more likely to feel a partnership with you and with the patient in getting through the illness or in managing it. Members of many Hispanic or Asian families in particular are often pleased to have something specific they can do for the patient, since in both cultures there is a long-held belief that illness in a family member involves the other family members as well. But no matter what their cultural origins, most patients feel the support and care received from their family as therapeutic and loving.

Take Time to Acknowledge Their Help

Be sure to give the family members or special friends some acknowledgment for what they do in support of the patient—particularly the ones who frequently come in with and seem to be looking after the patient. Try to make it something specific: "Mrs. Jones, these records of exactly when your husband took his medications are especially helpful to me, as well as to him, and I appreciate your thoroughness in checking this" or "Scott, your aunt is lucky to have your help getting here for her appointments. I know it would be difficult for her without your assistance. And I appreciate it too."

Caregiving family members need to be refueled occasionally. It's easy to become exhausted and stressed from the worry and effort of taking care of someone else, and simply run out of energy. Family members often feel tired, fearful, and guilt-ridden much of the time. It only takes a moment or two to reinforce their good efforts by a simple acknowledgment, and it can mean a great deal to them. This is particularly true when dealing with the family of elderly patients. "Most of us are inadequately prepared, emotionally and otherwise, to face the complex issues associated with caring for elderly loved ones" (Loverde, 2000, p. 3).

Let Family Members Know Your Feelings Too

Let your patient's family know that you have feelings about their loved one too. Let them see your interest and your sincere caring. When the physician assistant attending an elderly man tells him he won't be able to drive because of the medication he needs to take, it can help the patient as well as the family member if the physician assistant says, "I wish I didn't have to give you this news, and I'd much rather say you could still drive your car. The situation we're facing right now, however, requires this change."

If you indicate to the patient or patient's family that it is not easy for you to deliver the bad (or the not-so-good) news, it often helps them to know that you share their feelings. Your discomfort with imparting such news shows clearly that you have a caring relationship with the patient and with the family as a whole.

Make Your Patient Areas Family-Friendly

Have extra chairs (and perhaps fold-ups) in the exam room for family members. You may want to have one or two simple toys, a small set of blocks, or a box of crayons and paper for the children. They are less likely to see the entertaining and creative possibilities offered by your stethoscope or your blood pressure cuff. Small packets of fruit juice, perhaps the sort that comes in small boxes, can be handy for occasional treats or for patients who have been waiting too long. Extra diapers and tissue packets are also a thoughtful touch for waiting families.

Be sure to let them know where the nearest telephone is, or tell them they can use yours if that arrangement is manageable. Installing a pay telephone allows patients to make their calls without tying up your office phones. If you already have a pay phone, keep some coins handy for patients who might need them to make their calls.

KEEPING THE LINES OF COMMUNICATION OPEN

Knowing which family members to contact when the need arises is an important part of your overall care for your patients. Here are some suggestions and tips on how to do that effectively.

Ask Who the Main Contact Person Is

The direct approach is to simply ask the patient, if possible, whom he wants you to stay in contact with for updates and other information. Or you can have a meeting with the family, formally or informally as you think best, and ask them how they would like to handle the lines of communication. Perhaps they will want to choose one primary contact person and another as backup.

Determine the Leader

When a variety of people show up with the patient or contact you through long-distance telephone calls, it may be difficult to determine who is taking the leadership role or roles on behalf of the patient. Here are several approaches you can use to determine the family's leader and decision maker in these matters. It can be very important to you, to the patient, and to the family member(s) to establish a good working relationship right at the start and to nurture it as you go along.

The Influential Female

Very often it's the middle-aged female in the family who chooses you in the first place or is at least influential in the decision, as we mentioned in Chapter Two. She trusts you to take the best care of the patient, who may be her husband, parent, sibling, or child. If she feels you are not acting in the patient's best interest, or if she develops a strong dislike or distrust of you, chances are she will quickly find another clinician to take your place.

Introductions Can Indicate the Leaders

Sometimes the family members don't want to speak out about who holds a leadership position, or they can't agree as to who should be the main contact. Yet you may need to determine the leader or leaders in the group quickly. One way you might pick up important clues is through introductions. Ask for their names, as a basic courtesy rather than as a medical task, and their relationship to the patient. To start off the name giving, you can use a query that gets the patient involved: "And these are all members of your family?" This allows the patient to introduce them, often automatically introducing the leader or the most respected person first: "Yes, this is my father and my mother, this is my Uncle Jim, and these are my sisters, Clair and Beth."

Observe Body Language

You may also be able to determine who has the most influence in family matters from body language. The most powerful person often uses the least body language in reacting to you, less smiling or leaning forward, and lower facial affect. Also watch the body language of the group as a whole to see who they turn to or look at most often, especially when there is something important to consider.

Ask Who Stays

Another way you can determine who holds the leadership position among the family members accompanying the patient is by saying to the group, "We can only have two family members in the room at a time, and so I will have to ask the others to wait in the hall, just outside. Who will be staying?" As they make a group decision, you'll probably know who has the most influence by observing who makes the decision, and perhaps also by who stays.

Schedule a Family Telephone Time

Set aside a certain time each week when families know they can call you with any nonemergency questions they may have. Try to have a system worked out for information updates so that you don't have to say the same thing to each family member. This is where it comes in handy to know who the decision maker or the group leader is.

Actively Solicit Their Support

If you have a patient who is hospitalized, it may be helpful to ask the key family members for some additional support for that patient. You might telephone a key family member or members if you think your patient needs a little emotional uplifting. Ask for the person's assistance in helping the patient assume a positive attitude, explaining that this can sometimes make the illness or the recovery from surgery easier for the patient. Even if the family members cannot come into the hospital, an extra telephone call they make to their loved one can be very effective.

The family members often appreciate your efforts on the patient's behalf, especially in the area of emotional support. To avoid inadvertently sending the message that the family has not been attentive enough, be sure you begin by telling family members that their past support of the patient has been helpful and you therefore feel they will understand why you called to alert them that some extra support is needed at this particular time.

Telephone Distant Relatives Yourself

A helpful and caring approach that Lanny has used many times over the years is to ask his elderly patients' permission to call and talk to a son or daughter who lives out of town. This has proved to be tremendously helpful in reassuring the family and letting them know that their elderly loved one is being well cared for. Keeping adult children who live out of town informed is often a big relief to them; it tells them that you are making the extra effort not only on their behalf but on the patient's as well.

Suggest Community Resources

Keep a resource file of special support organizations in your community. Rather than recommending one specific group outright—OA (Overeaters Anonymous) for example—it might be a better idea to have a printed list of several support organizations in the community with a short description of their goals, their methods, and their services along with their phone numbers. This way, the patient or the family members can spot the organizations and support groups they think might be helpful and can then follow up if they are motivated to do so. If you suggest that a patient or family member might be helped by AA or Al-Anon (a support organization for families and friends of alcoholics) before you really know all the facts about the patient and the family members, they may be incensed by your implication. But if you include a comprehensive list of support groups along with other handouts, they can learn about this resource in a less threatening way.

Another resource in the community that can be especially helpful in counseling and supporting family members is the local clergy: ministers, rabbis, priests, and other clergy members, and those laypersons approved by the clergy for this support function. Lanny has often called on them, usually after getting family or patient approval first, to help families in times of medical crisis. Throughout his years of practice, these clergy members have often stepped in to ease patients' fears and sorrows and have ameliorated the families' emotional burdens as well. Their assistance also makes the physician's task more manageable.

Family Members Can Make Bad News Easier to Bear

If a patient needs to come in to talk with you about an upcoming procedure or for surgery, or to receive not-so-good-news, it can be helpful if a friend or family member comes along. If another person is there to hear the information, it can be useful later in following directions. It can also provide emotional support for the patient, who may be sad, fearful, or distraught by the end of the visit.

HOW TO DEAL WITH DIFFICULT FAMILY MEMBERS

Here are some specific strategies to deal with those hard-to-handle situations.

The Person Who Speaks for the Patient—Ceaselessly

One thing that irritates many clinicians is dealing with a spouse who has taken control of the situation—or perhaps has always been the controlling one—and wants to do the talking for the patient. We gave an example of dialogue on that topic and some insights in Chapter Three.

A scenario I have heard often from the physicians and other clinicians in the workshops centers on the family member who answers all the doctor's questions to the patient, and if the patient does squeeze in a few words, they are loudly discounted. "Harry, that's not so! You know you always have pains when you try to shovel the snow. Why do you tell the doctor that?! I tell him not to do it, doctor, but will he listen to me?" Sometimes the family member continues interjecting this way, generally taking the focus onto herself and requiring more time than might legitimately be needed for the visit. You have probably encountered family members of this sort.

There are times when you want to talk to the patient alone, as when you have to ask about elimination processes, sexual functioning, or other topics that could be uncomfortable for the patient to discuss in front of others. You

Communicating with Today's Patient

may sense that your questions might not be answered fully if another person is in the room. How do you get the family member to leave the examination room when you feel it's best for the patient? Whenever this topic comes up in the workshops, I suggest using some of the following techniques:

Instead of keeping your frustration in until you burst ("Look, I want to hear from the patient! You keep interrupting, and your husband never gets a word in edgewise here!"), we suggest you try using a three-part message:

1. State a benefit to the patient.

2. Say what you want or need.

3. Validate the family member.

It can go like this:

> Mrs. Collins, at this point, I think I can help your daughter more ... *(you are talking about the benefit to the patient)* if I can have some time alone with her *(you say what you want)*. Then it's *important* that I have an opportunity to talk to you again after that. So, be sure you stay nearby so we can have you come back in. *(This lets the family member know she is respected and seen as valued in this process, especially through the use of such words as* important *and* stay nearby. *It also lets her know she'll be coming back and is not just being dismissed.)*

Here's another example. Instead of saying curtly,

> If you keep asking questions, Mr. Joseph, I can't get anything done here! I think it would be better if you'd just wait outside—the nurse will bring you some magazines, and there's a TV you can watch. We'll call if we need you.

Try using this approach:

> At this point, Mr. Joseph, I need to examine your wife so we can get a better, more thorough idea of what we're dealing with *(you talk about the benefit to the patient—*better *and* thorough*)*. During

the examinations, we *do* need to ask you to wait outside. *(What you want: some private time with the patient as you do the examination and perhaps ask a few more questions without being interrupted.)* But it's also very important that I have an opportunity to talk with you a little later, so we'll be calling you back after we've finished the examination. *(Validation words he hears are very important and an opportunity to talk with you.)*

Keep in mind, this interpersonal dynamic of one person taking charge and the other being passive didn't just happen in your exam room. Although very ill people do tend to become more passive, it's likely that this is how these two people have related to each other for years. You probably can't change it, nor do they necessarily want you to. But you have to use skillful communications, such as the techniques we have described here, to deal with this type of situation so you can accomplish your medical tasks without incensing family members.

Send Body Language Signals About Who Talks When

Often you can get important information from the voluble family member that you might not get from the patient. Some clinicians like to have the talker remain in the room if they have a patient who is not forthcoming about symptoms. However, these clinicians also ask, "How can you get talkative relatives to be quiet for a while without asking them to leave?" Here's how.

Let's look in again on Harry and his wife: "Harry, that's not so! You know you always have pains when you try to shovel the snow. But will he listen to me?! Tell her, Harry; tell the doctor. And then he also has problems with sleeping, and he wakes up with terrible sneezing sometimes. I don't know why he won't tell you about it, but I'm right there and it wakes me up too. Tell her, Harry. . . ." At this point you probably want to jump in and say, "Be quiet so Harry *can* tell me!" But a better way would be to signal which person you want to hear from next, by turning your shoulders and upper torso toward that person.

First, turn your head and shoulders directly toward the talking family member, and respond briefly. Then turn your head and shoulders directly back toward the patient with an introductory phrase such as, "Well, I agree with your wife that I need to *hear from you* on this, (patient's name). So tell me, what has been *your* experience with these pains?"

Emphasis on the italicized words, coupled with the body language of an upper torso turn, signals the talkative family member that the focus has now shifted to the patient. Through your body language, your words, and your vocal intonations, you indicate who has the spotlight. This is a technique used by talk show hosts to control the speakers on a panel. Try it! I've used it to good advantage quite often.

Defusing the Irate Family Member

When angry family members come flying at you, it can be unnerving. You need to know quickly how to react. I suggest you use the techniques below to defuse the situation with any angry person you may encounter, but you will find the techniques especially helpful with angry and demanding family members.

1. Try to get them seated so you can all be at eye level as you listen to their complaint. If they are sitting, you sit down too. But if they prefer to stand, be sure you stand as well. If you do stand, get up slowly. Standing up suddenly can appear confrontational. Push your chair back first and then gradually straighten up.

2. Acknowledge their feelings. Nothing else is likely to be accomplished until you deal with the emotions involved. You can use a phrase such as "I can see you are upset about this, and I know your mother's comfort is very important to you."

3. Try to find something you can agree with. You might add here, "And I certainly agree with you. Her comfort *is* important!"

4. Then you can follow up with what you have to tell them.

Angry and demanding family members are likely to come to a receptive frame of mind if you avoid taking an immediately defensive position:

"Now look, Mrs. Green, one thing you have to realize is that we can't. . . ." This only serves to escalate the situation, in many cases.

If you get into a breakdown of communications during the rest of the conversation, try going back to the techniques we outlined above. Acknowledge their feelings, and find some area of agreement before you discuss the specifics of the problem—for example, "It's hard to be in pain and have to be poked at with needles for yet another blood test. I understand why you'd prefer your wife not have to go through that." Then give your explanation as to why the tests are essential.

It will also be helpful to take a moment to reread Chapter Three, on patient personalities, for additional tips on how to deal with strong, assertive personalities and also with people who may not tell you openly how angry they are—but find it easy to tell their attorney all about it later.

Don't Ignore Family Members

What happens if you brush off key family members? Plenty. Angry family members are often the ones who lodge complaints about the treatment of the patient, realizing that the patient may be too weak and too sick to fight with anybody about anything. Family members also speak out about the treatment *they* receive in the clinic or hospital. In addition, they tell their friends and, in some cases, the media.

What can you do to prevent this? Again, if you establish a caring and trusting relationship right at the start, with the patient and the significant friends and powerful family members, they will often overlook obstacles that may arise down the road.

The bottom line is that you always have to deal with family members and special friends of your patients. So those interactions might as well be positive—especially since these people close to your patient can wield a considerable amount of influence and are often consulted by the patient. As we've said, family and friends of your patients can be a great asset to you and can actually help you in achieving your goals with patients.

But perhaps most important is that a sizable body of research indicates quite clearly that patients do better if they have the loving support of friends and family around them. The benefits provided by many kinds of support groups for those who suffer chronic or terminal diseases have also been noted.

The support that friends and family can uniquely provide may be the most compelling reason of all to try to interact positively and effectively with patients' families and friends, even when they hurl their pent-up emotions at you instead of at the illness, which is often the real but unreachable target of their rage.

Years ago, I asked a friend, oncologist Chuck Denham, how he dealt with patients and family members who took out their anger at the disease on him. His reply was immediate and simple: "They're having so much pain and difficulty. I just try to love them through it."

Communicating with family members is a key aspect of treating a patient. They can play an important role in how well the patient adheres to the treatment plan, to the special diet, or to any other medical regimen you prescribe. A loving spouse or adult child can significantly influence your patient's compliance and the outcome.

A variation of this topic—communicating with patients and family members from other cultures—is the subject of the next chapter.

CHAPTER 9

Communicating Across Borders and Language Barriers

The health of the middle-aged Asian patient clearly has not improved. A few weeks earlier he was given medication that should have taken care of the situation. The puzzled physician asks if he has been taking the medication the way the prescribing doctor told him to. Yes, yes, he nods vigorously to assure her.

"Please show me exactly how you take the medicine," she directs. The patient reaches into his pocket and takes out the original prescription. It is carefully wrapped in waxed paper—barely legible—the writing blurred and runny, as if it has been left in the rain.

The patient asks for a glass of water. He then demonstrates his twice-daily routine: he puts the piece of paper with the prescription written on it carefully into a glass of water, and then he drinks the water. Carefully re-folding the dripping prescription in the waxed paper, he looks up with a quick smile and a nod of satisfaction.

He has done exactly what he was told when the doctor first handed him the prescription: "Here, take this with a glass of water twice a day."

Communication glitches such as these occur frequently, especially for clinicians who practice in large metropolitan areas where their patients come from diverse ethnic backgrounds. Even ordinary medical situations can present unexpected challenges because of cultural and linguistic differences. In this chapter, we suggest some techniques for dealing with the language barrier and with health beliefs and folk remedies that are often quite different from Western medicine (including various types of folk medicine) and that may affect your clinical interactions with these patients.

THE NEWEST AMERICANS

Today the largest wave of immigration since the early 1900s is changing the face of the United States. According to the U.S. Census Bureau (Schmidley and Gibson, 1999), more than fourteen million immigrants settled in the United States from 1981 to 1997. An even higher number of newcomers is projected for the period 1995 to 2025—approximately 20 million (Campbell, 1997).

Clinics and hospitals from Miami to Duluth to Los Angeles will reflect this mass influx. In recent years, most of the new immigrants have come from Mexico. The Philippines, China, Cuba, Vietnam, and India, in that order, are next in number of immigrants (Schmidley and Gibson, 1999). More than one-third of all newcomers are settling in California, with New York, Florida, New Jersey, and Illinois also receiving large numbers.

WHAT *MULTICULTURAL* MEANS

When we refer to cross-cultural or multicultural patients, it doesn't always mean immigrants. According to Marjorie Kagawa Singer, PhD., an anthropologist and nurse at the UCLA School of Public Health, *multicultural* means that the culture of the United States comprises many distinct groups, each with its own identity and integrity. These various subgroups interact constantly within the larger social structure, and they acculturate and assimilate to varying degrees.

As Kagawa Singer explains it, to assimilate is to give up one's native beliefs and values and take on those of the host country. Most immigrants assimilate enough to at least become bicultural. They adjust to the dominant culture, learning to function comfortably with its language, mannerisms, and values. But they can also live in the world of their ethnic or subcultural group with equal facility. Some prefer to minimize their interaction with the dominant culture and remain immersed in their subculture or ethnic enclaves.

Even people who have lived in the United States for many years—or who were born in the United States—and are fully acculturated may still carry on the beliefs, values, and behaviors of their native culture, or that of their parents' native culture, to some degree. Health beliefs and practices, therefore, may be the result of a blending of cultures.

ESTABLISHING THE RELATIONSHIP

In Chapter Two we discussed the importance of starting on a positive footing with your patients. When dealing with multicultural patients, some additional communication techniques may be helpful

Show Patients That You Are Interested in Their Culture

Gain patients' trust by showing an interest in their country, culture, and current events (while remaining sensitive to controversial political or economic issues). Ask a few questions to show that you are interested and nonjudgmental.

When you have patients from another culture, it can be quite interesting and educational to learn more about their homeland. Several resources that you might find interesting and helpful are listed at the end of this chapter. Notable among them is Culturegrams, an organizational spin-off from Brigham Young University.

Go Ahead and Use Your High School Spanish, But . . .

We encourage physicians who know a few words of a patient's first language to use them even if they are slightly mispronounced. Using their language shows your interest in patients and their country of origin. Using a few phrases or even conversing a little in their language early in the visit can build rapport and help the patient and the patient's family members feel relaxed.

But it's also important to realize that the level of foreign language required for chatting is far different from a thorough mastery of an entire language with all its subtleties. Proficiency is required to understand the patient's deepest health concerns and to give truly clear explanations. Once the small talk is over, try to find a qualified interpreter to help with the medical information.

Consider Family Support Important

In many ethnic groups, family support seems to be an integral part of all phases of the illness and recovery process. An efficient nurse or clinician who breezes in and quickly dismisses everyone but the patient may cause anxiety and may also be turning away the valuable assistance and psychological support provided to the patient by a nurturing and concerned family.

We suggest you ask large groups of relatives to select a few of the patient's closest relations to accompany the patient; then politely ask the others to wait in the reception room.

As mentioned in the previous chapter, whenever you are dealing with a group of relatives, we recommend that you ask them to help the patient once he or she returns home. They can perform a variety of useful tasks, such as changing bed linens, bringing water to the bedside, helping to monitor medications, and so forth. Helping the patient in this manner can provide an important ritual for the supportive family members in addition to practical assistance for the patient.

We're All Americans—North, South, and Central

Try to remember that people from countries south of the border often resent it when a North American says, "Well, here in America...."

"We come from America, too," they often point out. "South America, Central America, that's all America!" When referring to the United States, that's the term to use.

Communicating with Today's Patient

TECHNIQUES FOR TALKING OVER
THE LANGUAGE BARRIER

One physician who practices in a major metropolitan area and has many foreign-born patients tells us he often wishes he could see the conversations with patients from other cultures printed over their heads with annotated subtitles. That way, when he asks a question, he could see how his patient really interprets his words—and what the patient really means by his or her response.

We can't provide translations with annotated subtitles over patients' heads, but we can give you techniques that are helpful in communicating with patients from other cultures.

Slow Your Speech

Speak slowly, and add pauses. This gives the patient time to mentally translate as you go along. The technique discussed in Chapter Seven of pausing two beats between units of key information is particularly important for patients who speak limited English. For example, "Be sure to take this pill . . . two times a day, . . . one pill in the morning . . . and one pill at night, just before you go to sleep. . . ." If you give them too many words to digest, interpret, and react to, your patients may go quickly into information overload and simply shut down. They may nod politely but never tell you they didn't understand.

Use Clear Pictures or Diagrams

Pictures can be a great help. Patients welcome brochures with pictures and plenty of white space between the print passages, which makes the text easier to read and less intimidating. These brochures or other handouts can be taken home for additional study. Calendars are also useful for showing checked-off dates for return visits or procedures. Patients also appreciate the pictures and diagrams you draw yourself, if they are clear and easy to understand. Do this with care, because the drawing probably will be perused by all the patient's relatives.

Write Down Key Points

Write in large, easy-to-read print, using simple language. Write down essentials of the medications, and of course, write the name of the illness. Also write down the telephone number of the clinic so that the patient can ask about your written instructions if anything is not clear. Be sure that your name and telephone number are also printed legibly.

Ask Questions Many Ways

Ask specific questions, repeating them in different ways. Rephrasing your questions using alternative words gives patients another pass at understanding. They may know the translation of some but not all your words, so this rephrasing improves the chances that patients will understand you—if not the first time, then perhaps the second or third. Patients with limited English often won't admit that they don't understand and may smile and nod in agreement just to save face. Be careful not to raise your voice each time you rephrase or repeat. They are not deaf. Raising your voice may make your patients think you are angry.

Repeat Instructions and Verify Understanding

Have patients repeat your instructions as to how they will follow the treatment plan or medication routine before they leave your office or the hospital. You may even need to verify their understanding by asking them to demonstrate how they will do what you recommend—for example, taking a pill or using an inhaler.

Add Layers of Explanation from Other Experts

If you still suspect that the patient doesn't fully understand how to take the medication, you might arrange a conversation with a staff pharmacist or another local pharmacist to clarify or answer any additional questions the patient may have. This can be particularly helpful if the pharmacist speaks the native tongue of the patient. In Mexico, South America, and Central America, many people consult a pharmacist as readily as they do a physician. Pharmacists are allowed to dispense many medications without a physician's prescription, so foreign-born patients often are accustomed to visiting a pharmacist first to get medical advice and remedies, and may only go to a physician as a last resort.

Ask About Patients' Schedules

Eating and sleeping schedules of patients from other cultures may be quite different from yours. When you tell a patient to take a medication three times a day with meals, ask first, "When are your usual mealtimes?" In some cultures, breakfast may be eaten at midmorning, and dinner well after 8:00 P.M. Many Argentines and Europeans, for example, customarily eat dinner at about 9:00 or 10:00 P.M. or even later. A regular midday nap is important in many cultures—especially those originating in hot climates. So "bedtime" may be at midday and again at midnight for some patients.

Make Use of Interpreters

Today it isn't unusual for health care facilities to have interpreters on staff. Many hospitals are now required to provide interpreters for each foreign-speaking population that makes up a particular percentage of their census.

If doctor and patient don't share a common language, there is little hope of getting across the fine points of an illness or a treatment plan. Unless you work with a trained medical interpreter, it is almost impossible to have the level of communication necessary to assess and deal effectively with sensitive or complex health issues.

Try to find a qualified interpreter to help with essential medical questions and answers and with explanations of how to take medications. If you speak a little Spanish and your patient speaks a little English, you may think you have less need for an interpreter. But the language proficiency needed for giving clear explanations is far more than what you picked up on your trip to Puerto Rico two years ago. We recommend using an interpreter whenever possible in order to avoid serious problems due to misunderstanding.

For example, a twenty-five-year-old pregnant patient was told by her physician to take sitz baths for twenty minutes twice a day to relieve her symptoms of pain and swelling with immersion therapy. By the time the patient returned several weeks later, she had lost so much weight that an interpreter was called in. The patient was very proud to say that she'd faithfully taken her baths each day, even though they left her exhausted.

Wondering how bathing could be so tiring, the interpreter asked the patient exactly how she took her sitz baths. The woman described the process: she would get in the tub, then sit down, then stand up, sit down, stand up—over and over, for twenty minutes twice a day. Small wonder that she had lost so much weight and was feeling exhausted!

This situation could have been avoided if a professional interpreter had seen her on the first visit, explaining exactly the procedure for the baths, or if the patient had been required to repeat the instructions and demonstrate to the physician exactly how she would take her baths.

Be Careful About Guessing at Meanings of Words

It's easy to guess at meanings of words, and I admit to doing it myself. Several years ago, attending a function at the Argentine embassy, I was speaking with a small group of diplomats in my halting Spanish. I related an amusing story about an incident from earlier that day at the train station, which had left me feeling slightly embarrassed. Not knowing the word for embarrassed, I took a guess and said *embarrazada*. My listeners looked stunned; I had told them that as a result of the train mix-up, I was slightly pregnant.

One physician we spoke to on this topic said that while talking to a female patient he tried to explain that "It's not your fault." But he had to guess at the Spanish word for *fault*. He took a stab, used the English word, and simply added an *ah* sound at the end, saying, "Usted es sin faulta," which, to the patient, sounded like "You are without a skirt."

One Word Can Have Many Meanings

When speaking with a patient in a foreign language, be aware that words often have multiple meanings. As an example, consider how one word can have various meanings among the many regions of the Spanish-speaking world. There are multiple terms for "drinking straw." The word used for "throw up" does double duty as "bowel movement." It's tempting to guess at Spanish words, but doing so can have dire results.

If the patient comes in complaining of *susto* you might look it up in your Spanish-to-English dictionary and see that it means simply a sudden fright. To many from Mexico and other Spanish-speaking countries, this *susto* actually refers to something akin to posttraumatic stress syndrome, and many believe it can lead to serious complications, occasionally even resulting in death if not treated.

Your Message Is Taken Literally; Adjust for It

A young man from Southeast Asia, recently married to a young woman from the same region, came in to see the physician, saying that he wanted to use a condom for birth control. To demonstrate to the new husband how to apply the condom, the clinician had him hold out his forefinger and then showed him the correct way to unroll the device, carefully unfurling it down the patient's forefinger. The patient watched carefully, thanked the doctor, and left. But he was back a few months later asking why it hadn't worked—his wife was pregnant. The clinician asked the patient to describe exactly how he used the condom. As it turned out, the patient was using it faithfully, every night—on his forefinger.

It can be tempting to rush ahead and just do the translating yourself, especially when pressed for time. But trusting your memory of barely remembered high school foreign language classes or relying on the patient's relatives or friends can have serious consequences. It is best to use a qualified medical interpreter.

Using Family Members as Interpreters Can Backfire

When relatives are asked to translate, they may not transmit to you—or to the patient—any information that their culture deems inappropriate to discuss. If the topic includes reproductive organs or elimination processes, you'd be wise to use an interpreter. If a younger person—a son, daughter, niece, or nephew—is called on, he or she is likely to avoid such taboo topics, particularly with older relatives of the opposite sex. Translated information is apt to be misleading or incomplete because of their mutual embarrassment.

There is another serious problem inherent in using children as translators: in Asian, East Indian, and Hispanic cultures, among others, the hierarchy tends to be strict, with authority running from the male head of the family on down through the mother and older siblings. Traditionally, the head of the family is expected to make important decisions for other family members. If a child is suddenly in the higher-status position of interpreting for the father and his doctor, the family hierarchy is seriously disrupted, with the potential for increased stress on the patient and the child.

Miscommunication can also occur simply because the well-meaning patient or relative is confused about basic anatomy. We've been told often, for example, of foreign-born male patients citing as their chief complaint that they have pain in their vaginas. In one such case, a female relative had done the translating during an earlier visit.

Words that sound similar, such as "bladder" and "gallbladder," frequently are confused by patients and by relatives who are translating.

Giving Bad News

Don't assume that Hispanic or East Indian family members will give loved ones the news about terminal illness. Physicians who treat large numbers of patients from other cultures—Spanish-speaking ones in particular—often report that a family will plead with them not to tell the patient the bad news, for fear that openly stating a negative prognosis causes it to happen and thereby makes the patient worse.

Even if relatives do agree to translate the information, it is likely that the facts will be masked or significantly altered to protect the patient from bad news. Situations such as this require diplomacy and cultural sensitivity.

Meet with the Family

One technique is to call a special meeting with the family to discuss the issue. The physicians involved in the case can listen to the family's concerns about disclosing the information and can also explain why they think that gently revealing the reality of the situation is in the patient's best interest. This works out quite well in many instances. Be sure you present a caring and understanding manner during meetings of this sort.

TIPS ON NONVERBAL COMMUNICATION

How you present yourself can be just as important as how you present information. Generally speaking, your Asian and Hispanic patients prefer that you present a dignified, formal demeanor, because doctors are held in especially high esteem in their cultures. Using your first name, or theirs, is not recommended, nor is a jovial attitude. Hearty gestures such as back-slapping are considered inappropriate by Asian patients. To Japanese, for example, any broad gesture that uses the full or upper arm is considered impolite.

Social Distance

Social distance, known as "proxemics," differs widely among ethnic groups. Hispanic and Middle Eastern patients may want to sit or stand closer to you than you're accustomed to.

On the other hand, you'll find that many Asian patients prefer greater social distance—that is, sitting and standing farther away from you—as do many patients from Northern European backgrounds.

Touching

Mexican American patients tend to appreciate some appropriate touching during their medical visits, especially during examinations. For generations, therapeutic touching has played a significant part in the ritualistic treatments rendered by *curanderas* and other Mexican American folk healers (more on this later).

We recommend a handshake at the beginning of the medical interview, particularly for your male patients from other cultures. Key family members who have come with the patient for support also appreciate being acknowledged with a handshake. This can be especially important for patients from high-touch Hispanic and Mediterranean cultures.

We do not recommend a handshake for all cultures or all patients, however. Women who have recently immigrated from many of the Asian countries, for example, would probably prefer that you not shake hands. Cultures in which male and female behavior are highly differentiated are also less likely to encourage female handshaking. Most Asian patients and northern European-born patients tend to prefer less touching and a more formal approach generally than do Mexican American, South American, and Central American patients and those from Mediterranean areas.

Same-sex hugging or handholding is common in many cultures, and it is not a sign of homosexuality. Arab men commonly hold hands as a sign of male friendship. Male friends in Italy, Argentina, and other parts of South and Central America give an *abrazzo*, a mutual side-to-side hug upon meeting, while their wives often greet each other by kissing the air as they touch both cheeks. Korean women and girls often hold hands as they walk together.

It's advisable not to pat Asian children on the head, even though this is a common gesture of affection in the United States. Among Southeast Asians in particular, the head is thought to be where the spirit dwells and is deserving of special respect.

Finally, if you must use an otoscope to look into the child's ear, use a tongue depressor to look into the mouth, or insert a needle into a scalp vein to give an infant intravenous infusion, we recommend that you begin by telling the parent what you are about to do and why it is necessary and beneficial for the child. Many Southeast Asians—especially Laotians—believe that the spirit can be released from the orifices of the head, thereby resulting in serious illness or even death.

SPECIFIC BODY LANGUAGE THAT MAY CAUSE PROBLEMS

Following are two areas where problems can easily arise.

Hand Gestures

To you, a beckoning hand gesture made with the upward curl of the fingers may mean only "Come on up onto the table, and let's have a look at you." But it can be taken as a serious insult by a patient from another culture. That's how one calls a dog or other animal in Southeast Asia. Instead, people are beckoned with the palm facing downward and the fingers moving in downward curling strokes.

Our common "Come here" hand gesture, with palm up and the first finger curling toward oneself, is how a prostitute is beckoned in parts of the Philippines. Similarly, the positive "thumbs-up" gesture commonly used here is an insult to Nigerians and Australians.

More lewd than rude is the familiar OK sign made with the thumb and forefinger forming a circle. A well-meaning "It's great that the medication seems to be helping," when accompanied by this gesture, can leave your patients from Argentina, Brazil, Russia, or Germany scowling and shocked at your obscenity.

Eye Contact

Eye contact varies by culture. Koreans, Filipinos, and many other Asian groups, as well as Native Americans, consider direct eye contact rude and confrontational; among East Indians and many Asians it often has sexual connotations as well.

When discussing eye contact and cultural differences in one of our workshops, a physician who had practiced in the Pacific Islands with a large medical corporation realized why he had been so frustrated in trying to communicate with his young patients. "I felt irritated because they wouldn't look me in the eye," he said. "Sometimes I'd lean over and turn my head almost upside down to see their faces, to get some kind of reaction to what I was saying." Since he was a large man, this contorted position was especially uncomfortable and probably made his patients even more so.

He was pleased to learn that the children's culture viewed their lack of eye contact as a sign of respect for him, as well as good manners. This attitude about eye contact and respect is shared by many from other cultures as well.

A dramatic example of how nonverbal communication, specifically eye contact coupled with touch, can affect multicultural patients occurs in what is referred to as *mal de ojo*, or evil eye. Picture yourself in this scenario. A Mexican American family, still tied closely to beliefs of the Mexican countryside, comes to your clinic. The young mother is the patient; she has a mild upper respiratory infection. She is holding her young child, whom you acknowledge with a simple "What a pretty baby" or other ordinary phrase. You continue the examination; the mother is treated and everyone leaves.

Two days later you receive a telephone call from an unhappy father, who claims that the baby is very ill because you put a curse on him—*mal de ojo*. You insist that all you did was pay a passing compliment; you never even touched the child.

That's the problem. If you had touched the child while looking at him admiringly, you would not have put the curse on him, according to folk medicine beliefs in Mexico (particularly in rural areas). Now the family must bring the baby, sick with vomiting and fever, back into the clinic, and you must touch him to remove the curse.

A simple way many physicians avoid such situations is by lightly touching the Mexican American patient's child or children as they acknowledge them in the examining room.

Often just an appropriate light touch on the hand, arm, or back of the head is enough to ensure that you won't be seen as putting as a curse on them.

RECOGNIZING SIGNS OF COMMON FOLK REMEDIES

A patient may not always be willing to tell you that he is using folk medicine. Not knowing this can lead to misunderstanding.

Is It Folk Medicine or Child Abuse?

Among Southeast Asians, a procedure using a small Pyrex-like, bell-shaped glass jar—a "Giac cup"—is believed to remove unwanted elements from the body. One woman in the community is usually the "cupper," carefully trained by the previous cupper. A cotton swab at the end of a stick is dipped in alcohol, set alight, and then inserted into the cup. Oxygen is absorbed as the air inside the cup heats; the cup is quickly placed, with the opening downward, on the skin, usually in the chest or upper back area. As the air inside the cup cools, the skin is pulled up slightly into the cup. This cupping is often done again and again, with several cups covering the area at the same time.

Cupping was used as a home remedy for many generations in parts of Russia and France. It is still used in some areas of those countries, we are told. Although not normally painful to the patient, this procedure often leaves reddened circular marks on the skin that have been misinterpreted frequently by clinicians as evidence of spouse or child abuse.

Another common folk remedy used by Southeast Asians is *cao gio*, or "coining." An oil containing eucalyptus is applied to the skin; then the rim of a coin is rubbed gently against the skin until ecchymotic striations appear on the skin. These stripes of dark blood under the skin can often be observed in parallel stripes down the arm or the back. It's believed that this procedure relieves pain. Vietnamese and Hmong patients we have interviewed say that coining is not a painful procedure, and they believe it to be effective. When seen in hospitals and clinics, however, these dark stripes have also been misinterpreted as evidence of child or spouse abuse, occasionally resulting in police reports and embarrassing confrontations.

Use Open-Ended Questions to Find Out About Folk Remedies

Once you have established some trust and confidence, ask open-ended questions such as, "What have you been doing to take care of these symptoms?" or "What other home remedies have you been using?" Patients are more apt to tell you important information with these open-ended questions.

There is much more to be said about multicultural communication, including the theories of "hot" and "cold" foods and remedies, concepts of the locus of control of illness, the ancient belief in the four elements, and other aspects of the health care beliefs of various cultures. However, we have touched on some of the main points for dealing with patients from other cultures, which we hope will be helpful.

In areas with a high concentration of people from Spanish-speaking countries, there are often folk healers such as *curanderas* and *curanderos*. These folk healers use an assortment of religious and mystical symbols plus therapeutic touching and sometimes even hypnosis to help their patients. Your patients may be seeing both you and a folk healer at the same time. Or they may be using herbal teas, for example, that can interfere with some medications, so it is important to find out what other measures the patient is taking to heal a particular illness.

If your patients do tell you about other folk remedies they are using, be sure you listen with respect. Rolling the eyes or hisses of "can-you-believe-this," even under your breath, are clearly out of place and disrespectful of the patient and the patient's culture. We have had foreign-born physicians in our workshops tell us that even though, as physicians, they know some of the folk remedies their mothers used are not scientifically proven to be beneficial, they nevertheless go back to these remedies, often self-administering them when they are really ill. They admit to doing this for the comfort and the memories of being lovingly taken care of that these folk remedies bring back to them.

One final word of caution: It is easy to oversimplify the topic of multicultural communications. Don't assume that all ethnic groups are homogeneous or monolithic in terms of their beliefs and behaviors. Each patient is still unique and not a stereotype of his or her culture. It is essential to elicit individual health beliefs and practices, since factors such as socioeconomic status and length of time in the United States can make a significant difference. None of us want to be stereotyped when we travel abroad, and neither do patients who come here from other regions of the world.

Here's a good example as to how cultural stereotyping might feel. The next time you begin treating a patient from another country, picture yourself in this scenario.

You're traveling in Hungary. You become ill and go to a Hungarian clinic. The doctor doesn't speak much English, but he has read a few articles about the United States. To help with the language barrier, the doctor asks one of the patients out in the waiting room who speaks a little English to come in and translate his questions for you.

The questions go like this: "Do you believe your health depends on the doses of vitamins you are taking?" "Like most people in the United States, you probably think that this illness is caused by too much stress, eh?" "You mentioned that you're from California, so I suppose you will want some crystals to gaze at for your health and some herbal teas, right?"

Given the dramatic increase in immigrants to the United States, it is essential for physicians to be more aware of the sensitivity and respect needed to treat multicultural patients, and to be cognizant of the complexities that may be involved.

OTHER RESOURCES

Finally, here are two resources that may be useful in learning about multicultural patients:

1. *Culturegrams* are a series of four-page newsletters, one for each of 130 countries, that provide easily digestible information on customs and courtesies, the people, lifestyles, the nation, and references for additional study. You can obtain copies by calling (800) 528-6279 or by writing to Culturegrams at 1305 North Research Way, Orem, UT 84097.

2. *Honoring Patient Preferences: A Guide to Complying with Multicultural Patient Requirements*, by Anne Knights Rundle, Maria Carvalho, and Mary Robinson (eds.), San Francisco: Jossey-Bass, 1999. This book includes brief, easy-to-follow descriptions of the key communication styles and critical cultural beliefs for many ethnic and lifestyle groups.

We've covered numerous communication topics so far: greeting patients, working with various personality types, body language, listening skills, and dealing with patients' family members. We now turn to one last topic: what your overall professional image communicates to your patients.

CHAPTER 10

Shining Up Your Professional Image

"Oh, please don't let that be the new doctor!" Joan whispers to her husband as a young woman carrying charts walks past. The older couple are making their first visit to a new primary care physician. Recently retired to Tucson, Joan has chosen her doctor, sight unseen, from a list sent by their new health care plan.

The young woman, in a white jacket, is also wearing a full, ankle-length, black lace skirt; platform high heels; and rhinestone drop earrings that waggle brightly as she walks. Her hair, an unnaturally bright color, swirls in high piles on top.

Doug quickly retorts, "You mean you'd base your judgment of a doctor's training and medical abilities on something as superficial as how she's dressed?"

Joan looks sheepish, thinks a moment, and then straightens up and shoots back: "Yes! Actually, I *do* make conclusions about her based on how she looks. Anyone who can profoundly affect my life should have good judgment—be able to make sensible decisions. That young woman showed poor judgment from the time she woke up this morning and decided what to wear today. If that's the doctor, I'm out of here. I'll wait in the car."

DO'S AND DON'TS FOR APPAREL CHOICES

Appropriate dress for physicians and other clinicians is part of your professional image and is usually learned informally from a variety of sources.

221

Studies at Brigham and Women's Hospital in Boston and H. C. Moffett Hospital in San Francisco found that many of the staff physicians had dress habits that were less formal than what most of their patients preferred (Dunn and others, 1987).

The term "business casual" has, in more recent years, become a fashion trend. "Casual Fridays" are observed in corporations throughout the nation—although there are some indications that this casualness in dress may be shifting back again to a more conservative look.

Here, we cover some general guidelines for appropriate professional attire, but there is no easy answer to the specifics. Thousands of years ago, Hippocrates described the physician as "clean in person, well-dressed and anointed with sweet-smelling unguents" (Jones, 1923). Things haven't changed a whole lot in that respect—except for the unguents.

Patient Expectations

Today's patients seem to have something of an internalized template in their minds of what a doctor, or any health care professional, should look like, just as Joan has. The closer you come to fitting this template, the more readily you gain patients' trust and confidence.

What you wear, how you are groomed, and how your office looks are all indications of your professional values. These are also silent messages you transmit about your practice, messages that can make or break a relationship with a patient. When asked by researchers if their confidence in the ability of a doctor was based on the doctor's appearance, 41 percent of patients in one study said yes (McKinstry and Wang, 1991). The male doctors who were identified by patients as "more believable" were wearing white coats or sports jackets, plus shirts and ties. The female physicians selected as more believable were wearing white coats and simple blouses and skirts.

Your professional image may also affect not only patients' confidence in you but also their adherence, since whether patients follow your medical advice often depends on their assessment of your clinical knowledge and your judgment.

White Coats

Several studies have looked at whether patients prefer clinicians in white coats or in more casual attire (McKinstry and Wang, 1991). Patients do tend to prefer white coats, whether the clinicians are male or female, and they tend to prefer clinicians who dress traditionally or conservatively.

In recent years, the white coat has been doffed by many pediatricians and others who deal with children because of the widespread perception among health care professionals that a white coat is intimidating to children. However, some studies say otherwise, indicating that pediatricians can wear white coats without fear of jeopardizing their relationships with pediatric patients, even with children as young as four to eight years old (Matsui, Cho, and Rieder, 1998).

In addition, both parents and children tended to view informally dressed physicians negatively; both assessed them as less competent than physicians dressed conservatively. Parents tended to feel more strongly about it, however, than their children (Marino, Rosenfeld, Narula, and Karakurum, 1991).

When pediatrician Andrea Houfek attended our workshop several years ago, I recommended she wear her white coat when seeing patients. Several months later, in an article in *Medical Economics* that listed some of the benefits clinicians derived from Desmond Medical Communications workshops, Dr. Houfek was quoted: "I'm fairly young and I'm female and that doesn't tend to make a lot of people respect you. I never used to wear a white coat because I felt it would scare the children, but I started wearing the coat and the kids don't seem to notice. From parents—particularly older women—I've found that I get a very different response. I feel they think more of me based on their first impression. Now, there's no more confusion over who's the doctor and who's the nurse" (Bell, 1995, p. 48).

When you put on your white coat, be sure it is clean, with no dirt or stains on it. Be sure also there are no pocket corners coming off or seams coming open, especially under the arms.

Other Good Apparel Choices

Patients had other clothing preferences in addition to the white coat. Many who responded to surveys of attire for physicians indicated that female physicians wearing skirts and simple professional blouses are dressed more appropriately than are those wearing trousers. Unfortunately the researchers did not look at the attitudes of patients regarding female clinicians wearing suits, which we think is a perfectly reasonable option and, depending on the suit, entirely professional.

For men, a solid or tweed jacket or a suit, combined with a conservative shirt and tie, consistently received the highest approval ratings from the patients queried. Blue jeans and beach shorts brought high levels of disapproval, as might be expected.

Patterns and Prints

When choosing shirts, dresses, or blouses, avoid large block plaids or large floral prints, particularly if they are in bright, bold colors. These are probably not conservative enough for a health care setting. Stick with conventional, quiet prints or patterns. Big-and-bold looks as if you are trying to attract attention to yourself. Avoid using more than two of the three basic patterns: stripes, geometrics, or florals. Three can make your overall image too "busy."

Colors

Friendly, unintimidating colors are browns, tans, lighter blues and blue-grays, burgundies, soft golds or yellows, and other warm and optimistic colors in medium tones. These are colors that make you appear approachable and comfortable to be around.

Avoid wearing shirts or blouses that are very dark or drab, such as dark gray, drab olive green (unless you are a redhead), or black. Avoid wearing a dark shirt with a dark tie or scarf. Such somber colors can leave an ominous sense of "bad news" in your patients' perceptions.

Cool and Breezy

Choose natural fabrics, such as wool, cotton, silk, or blends of these. Natural fabrics breathe better than synthetics such as nylon and polyester, which are often uncomfortable as temperatures rise. You will feel more relaxed in natural-fiber clothing, especially when you are rushed or stressed. In addition, these fabrics often have a better "hand," which means they hang better and hold their shape. Higher-quality clothing is often made using these natural, nonpolymer-based fibers.

There is one caveat about wearing natural fibers such as cotton and linen: be careful about wrinkling. It's important to wear outfits that look crisp and neatly pressed. A colleague tells of a woman who decided against a particular plastic surgeon for her facelift when she saw his wrinkled suit. If the surgeon thought his suit good enough to wear in this professional setting, she wondered what he would consider good enough for her face!

Collars

If you wear shirts that button up to the neck, be sure your shirt collar is the right size. As men age and add or lose weight, they often continue wearing a shirt collar size that fit in earlier years but no longer does.

Be certain also that your collar is neat and flat. A collar that is wrinkled or askew sends the message that you may not be precise, may not take time to be careful and thorough. The collar is close to your face, so it is easily observed by the patient. A collar that is too tight or too loose is unattractive and can give the impression of carelessness.

"T'd" Off

Is it even necessary to mention that T-shirts that have sexually suggestive sayings imprinted on them, phrases that disparage people from diverse populations, or other offensive sayings have absolutely no place in the professional setting of health care? We would have thought not, except that three health care professionals have shown up in our patient communication workshops over the years wearing these tops. Besides the poor attitude conveyed through the message on the shirt, an even louder message is being sent about the lax management of a health care organization that allows such unprofessional attire.

Modesty

This may also seem an obvious message, but having had to counsel clinicians on a number of occasions regarding modesty in their choice of apparel, we think it worth mentioning here. Any clothing that draws overt attention to your sexuality is distracting to patients (as well as to coworkers). Over the years, a number of female clinicians have worn outfits into our workshops that included tight sweaters, tops that showed cleavage, or blouses that hung open as the clinician leaned forward. In addition, we have observed skirts that were too short or too tight and pants that were too form-fitting, all of which were inappropriate in any professional setting. Male clinicians should avoid tight pants as well as shirts worn open at the neck, particularly if this exposes any chest hair.

A young female pediatrician arrived in one of our California workshops a few years back wearing a noticeably short, tight miniskirt. She giggled that parents often looked at her in surprise and said, "Oh, are *you* the pediatrician?" Later, during the course of the workshop, she mentioned that parents often didn't seem to listen to her or follow her advice. Well?

Scrubs

Scrubs are appropriate in emergency room and urgent care settings or in a surgical area of a hospital, if needed. But the preferred style for a clinician, when meeting patients in the office, is still a traditional shirt, tie, and white coat or jacket for men and a white coat or jacket with skirt and blouse for women.

Because health care is a conservative profession, when deciding on your wardrobe, choose optimistic colors and current styles, but keep them tastefully restrained, uncluttered, and neat. If you are not sure about an outfit or accessories, consider the old folk wisdom: "When in doubt, leave it out."

Practice What You Preach

Your advice to patients to eat a healthy diet, get plenty of exercise, and have a healthy lifestyle will be more convincing if you set the example and model the behavior you want to encourage in patients. Shedding any extra pounds and working out regularly will keep you looking fit and capable, important to your professional image.

ACCESSORIES

Accessories are often designed to catch the eye. Choose them with care so that they don't distract from what you are saying or misrepresent you in any way.

Ties

Ties received a very high approval rating in all the surveys of patient preferences in attire for clinicians. An overall conservative print or regimental striped tie is usually a good choice, preferably with some warm yet conservative colors such as burgundy or muted gold. Avoid any wild prints or boldly contrasting colors. Save that bold tie with faces of your favorite rock group, or the one with the hundred dollar bills printed all over it, for Saturday night (assuming you're not on call).

What's appropriate and what isn't depends to some extent on where you practice, who your patients are, and how long they've known you. If you live in an area such as Phoenix, where it is customary to wear, say, a bolo tie with a turquoise nugget at the top, this may be an entirely appropriate tie for you to wear into the clinic or hospital. It is probably not suitable if your practice is in Duluth or New York City.

Jewelry

Avoid wearing too much jewelry, especially jewelry that clanks, clatters, or jiggles. Avoid clunky watches or bracelets that rattle against the desk as you write in the chart, as well as oversized rings, real or knock-off Rolexes, and any other jewelry that draws attention or connotes wealth.

Women's earrings should be conservative. Anything larger than a quarter is probably too large for the health care setting. Avoid dangling earrings that swing back and forth. These tend to demean your authority and distract your patient's attention from the medical information. No rhinestones or other shiny stones. These are appropriate only for evening wear.

Male clinicians should think carefully about wearing an earring. When queried, 55 percent of patients in Great Britain said they would not approve of a male physician wearing such jewelry (McKinstry and Wang, 1991).

Cartoon Characters

Accessories such as ties, wrist watches, or scarves with cartoon characters are fine for those who work exclusively with children. Many pediatricians and pediatric nurse practitioners like to wear ties or scarves with cartoon characters cavorting about on them.

Eyeglasses

Glasses with thick rims, especially those with very dark rims (or with white or silver-colored plastic rims), can make you appear owlish. They can also be intimidating, setting up a barrier between you and the patient. Instead, wear standard-size, conservative rims that neither attract attention nor distract your patient from listening to your medical advice.

Avoid half-glasses. Although they are stylish, they also encourage a kind of peering-over head position, which can be intimidating to patients. Avoid "cat-eyes" styles or glasses with fancy swirls at the corners of your glasses, particularly those with rhinestones added.

Shoes

Avoid open-toed sandals, clogs, or sneakers. These are too informal for the medical environment. Studies show that patients generally prefer conservative and professional-looking footwear. Platform heels or any very high heels are also inappropriate, even if you have an important personal occasion right after work. It's difficult to walk around a busy clinic or medical office in those all day, anyway.

Athletic shoes—such as tennis, aerobic, or running shoes—are increasingly used in hospital settings, especially in urgent care, and are acceptable in that area, since rubber-soled shoes are safer than conservative leather-soled shoes when one has to run on slippery floors. Those who work in a hospital are generally on their feet all day, and the new walking or training shoes may keep energy and comfort levels higher. But there is still some mixed opinion as to the appropriateness of such athletic shoes when seeing patients in your office.

Don't Leave Home Without Your Badge

Whatever apparel choices you make, there is one item patients really like to see you wear: a badge bearing your name. Wear your name badge just above the upper pocket on your white coat, with your name appearing in letters large enough that most patients can read it without eyeglasses. You can put the badge on either side of your jacket. We favor the right side for right-handed people because as you shake hands with a patient it is where they can most readily read your name. Clinicians who are left-handed may also prefer to wear the badge on the right side, since this is still where most patients are likely to look for it.

In today's health care setting, where a variety of health care professionals see patients, it is especially important to wear a badge that has your name and an indication as to whether you are a physician assistant, nurse practitioner, physician, or other type of health care professional.

GROOMING

Hairstyles

Ponytails, on men or women, connote a degree of youthfulness. You may be thought of as less mature and be taken less seriously by some patients if you choose to wear your hair this way.

Your hairstyle should not require rearranging while you are in front of patients. I have had young physicians in our workshops, both male and female, who wore long, blond "surfer-dude" tresses that needed to be flopped back regularly from the front of the face. This can be very distracting and irritating to anyone who is talking with you and may even seem

Shining Up Your Professional Image

unhygienic. It also appears youthful and can make you seem a bit self-absorbed. Avoid any hairstyle that might need to be adjusted while you are talking with the patient.

Avoid preening your hair as you listen to or talk to your patients. Patting your hair, even at the back of the neck, or twisting or twirling a section of hair around your finger can be read by patients as your being nervous, or even flirtatious.

Be careful of long bangs or hair that hangs down in front of your eyes. This can make you appear untrustworthy. It can also look sloppy or "geekish," as if you are hiding behind your hair. Your eyes need to be easily and fully seen by the patient.

On Your Face

A well-groomed mustache or a groomed beard are fine and even considered traditional (especially with the example set by Dr. C. Everett Koop). Patients generally seem to rate beards and mustaches favorably (Matsui, Cho, and Rieder, 1998).

Makeup and Perfume

Women's makeup should be subtle and understated—but there! A little color in the face adds interest and vitality. Be careful that your makeup is neither too flashy or brightly colored nor too dark or heavy. For example, avoid thick mascara on the eyes.

A clinician in one of our California workshops wore dark brown lipstick, a current fad at the time, which made her look as if she had a liver disease. To a three-year-old patient, it would probably look scary or witch-like, and to a sixty-three-year-old patient absurd and inappropriate. Save any current makeup fashion trends for the weekend, when you're with your own age group.

Earlier in this chapter we cited Hippocrates and his recommendation of anointing with unguents. On that topic, try to avoid any perfumes or aftershave lotions that have a noticeable aroma. Heavy, flowery perfumes worn by women or strong-smelling aftershave or colognes worn by men are distracting and generally considered unprofessional. They may also seem flirtatious to some patients.

Nails

A standing appointment with a good manicurist is recommended—once a month at least—to keep nails clean and clipped. Women's nails should be no longer than just cresting above the top of the finger. Nails that grow to be very long can easily be seen by patients as potential breeding places for germs, and they are not professional looking.

If you are wearing nail polish, be sure it is a simple, subtle tone. Do not wear appliqués on the nails, such as tiny fruits, flowers, or gold initials. They are inappropriate for anyone in health care, including those at the front desk. If your polish wears off, even partially, redo it before you see patients. A phlebotomist in a clinic we worked with had long, dirty nails with partially worn off nail polish that was garish orange. Patients don't want someone with fingernails like that touching them, much less inserting needles into their veins. Her hands and grooming called into question the clinic's overall standards of cleanliness and professionalism.

Grooming in Public

All personal grooming should take place in private or in the lavatories. Those who work in your office should be reminded of this too. Personal grooming, such as combing or brushing the hair, using a toothpick, or flossing, is never good manners in public or in the professional setting. It can be offensive to patients who are exposed to this kind of behavior as they wait in the reception area.

Cleanliness

Washing your hands or changing your gloves in the patient's view is highly recommended by our colleague Susan Keane Baker. In her book *Managing Patient Expectations* (1998, p. 39), she suggests that if you don't have a sink in the examining room, you can ask a staff member to tell the waiting patient, "Dr. Jones will be right in. She's just washing her hands." Baker advises those caring for patients to be "conspicuously obvious" in following standard precautions as a way of reducing the anxiety that patients may feel about cleanliness or transmission of contagious diseases.

YOUR OFFICE IMAGE

The general environment that your patients observe in your reception area and in your exam or treatment rooms can send important messages about your practice.

Comfortable and Neat

Your office should be neat, orderly, and attractive in a professional, comfortable, and understated way. A messy, cluttered office indicates to patients that you may also have a messy, cluttered mind. Dirt and dust accumulated in corners may be associated in your patient's mind with your overall attitude toward personal hygiene and cleanliness. Piles of patient files should be put where they belong. There should be absolutely no visible signs of blood anywhere, not even in or on top of waste cans. Waste cans, by the way, should have covers that open by foot pedal.

Framed Pictures and Credentials

We do like to see a few academic awards framed conservatively and hanging on the wall. Patients like them as well, although these academic credentials are often not as important to patients as the smile and look of interest on your face while you're talking with them.

One family portrait in your office is fine, if your group or organization allows it. In fact, it can help put a positive light on you as a loving parent, husband, wife, or partner. We do not recommend, however, a whole collection of photos; one or two medium-sized portraits of your loved ones is sufficient.

Bulletin Boards

Avoid bulletin boards loaded with photos that are pinned up at odd, haphazard angles, overlapping postcards from family and friends, yellowing newspaper cartoons, and children's' drawings dangling off the edges of the bulletin board. This looks more like a kid's clubhouse or the front of someone's refrigerator than a professional office that deals with major health issues.

If your practice caters to the pediatric population, by all means put up the pictures and cards they send. We suggest, however, that you put them in one or two particular areas set aside for just that purpose. Keep the display looking neat, as well as fun and enjoyable, with all pictures arranged generally within the edges of the frame. The same goes for cartoons; a few neatly displayed cartoons are OK, but none with ragged edges from having been torn out of the newspaper and none that are yellowed by age. Of course, be cautious of cartoons that use biting sarcasm as their form of humor. Avoid humor based on political, religious, gender, or ethnic topics. Patients may not find these amusing.

Reading Material

Periodicals, including popular magazines and newspapers, should be current—nothing older than three or four months. In addition, they should cover a range of interests and reflect, if possible, your patient base. If you practice in a middle-class suburb of a large city and have many young families among your patients, you would probably include some magazines specifically on child care. If your practice serves largely professional people, the newspapers and magazines that pertain to business might be more appropriate. And if you are in an inner-city location, the publications in your reception area should reflect the interests of that patient base as well.

Be sure to have a stack or even a rack of pamphlets on health information for patients to read. These should be in the reception area and also in the exam rooms for patients to read while they wait for you.

Front Desk Access

If you have a glass or plastic panel that slides open and closed at the front desk, advise your staff about its proper use. The panel should never be quickly shut while a patient is still standing in front of the desk. Staff should shut this panel only after the patient has been seated. It is rude to hand a patient forms to fill out or referral papers and then quickly slide the panel shut. Be sure also that such panels are not frosted so that the patient cannot see in. This creates a barrier to those who may want to speak with or ask a question of someone at the desk.

Waiting Patients

Your staff should check in on any patient who has been waiting longer than fifteen minutes. They should apologize for the delay and see if that patient needs to telephone anyone, since the person will be leaving the medical visit later than expected. They can offer reading material and perhaps a small container of fruit juice if it is near a meal time.

No Food Aromas

Many staff lounges in clinics and hospitals and the break rooms of medical offices are equipped these days with microwave ovens. Packets of popcorn and other microwavable foods offer quick, filling lunches for busy clinicians and office staff. But the cooking odors of these foods waft far beyond the area of the staff lounge or break room, penetrating into the patient areas (waiting rooms, exam rooms, hospital rooms).

The aroma of popcorn is more suited to a movie matinee than a medical office, and pizza aromas more to a bowling alley or restaurant than a clinic or hospital. Some patients may remark jokingly about these food odors, but others who are ill can become nauseous; those who are fasting are likely to be irritable and uncomfortable. The aroma of popcorn or any other cooked food is inconsiderate and unprofessional; it sends a message of a too-casual attitude. Just as heavy perfumes and aftershave lotions are not appropriate odors in the serious, disciplined medical environment, neither are food odors—even if it is a staff member's birthday.

Also, be aware that it is never appropriate to eat or drink in any area where patients might see you doing so.

Using the Telephone

No one in your office or clinic should be conducting a private telephone conversation while a patient is in the area, certainly not if the patient is waiting in front of them as they talk on the phone.

No chewing of any sort should be done while talking on the phone with patients or patients' families. The sounds of chewing food or gum are readily picked up on the phone, and this is always rude and much too casual. In fact, there should be no gum chewing in the professional medical environment—*ever.*

Finally, patients have expectations as to how a medical office, clinic, or hospital should look, just as they have a general idea in their minds of how a clinician should look (as Joan did). The closer you come to matching or fulfilling the popular concept, the easier it is for you to have good relations with your patients and with the family members who come with them. It doesn't take any more of your time to have a professional image that sets the stage for greater likelihood of positive communication between you and your patients.

CONCLUSION

During times of change, we all occasionally need a stepped-up dosage of motivation. As a busy clinician, you are faced with myriad new requirements and a daily stream of patients, some of them challenging and taxing. If you are like the clinicians we see in our patient communication workshops throughout the nation, you probably need to be reminded from time to time of the significant social value of what you do, and the importance of the skills and knowledge you bring to your practice. One of our goals in this book has been to give you such a reminder.

As Lanny observes,

The medical profession is unique. During our long educational process, we all experience the science that medicine is based upon. By training, we're analytical, and we're taught to use this type of thinking when approaching the problems of the patients we care for.

To me, what makes medicine unique is that, although steeped in science, it also requires us to interact with patients—each with their very own personality. To relate to patients, we must be able to communicate with them so they can tell us what concerns them. Anyone who has had patient contact knows this can be very difficult.

Yet it's just this that makes the profession so rewarding. If practicing medicine consisted only of the scientific aspects, it would not be enjoyable. But taking the time to get to know individual patients and how they react to their health problems—that is what makes it worthwhile and gratifying.

We both clearly remember our own family doctors' house calls. Despite growing up in different parts of the country, we recall that things seemed to improve—everyone just felt more relieved—as soon as the physician stepped through the door. Our family doctors seemed to carry something special along with their black bags: an aura of knowledge, kindly understanding, and a way of talking with us that showed their sincere interest. We have occasionally discussed how our own family physicians, Dr. Henry Conrad and Dr. Ralph diCosola, influenced us in our choice of health care professions. These early impressions have, at some level, also been an underlying inspiration throughout our work on this book.

Although much has changed in health care, some things remain constant. Your professional satisfaction is still affected by your day-to-day communications with patients; conversely, your communications with patients are profoundly influenced by your degree of professional satisfaction. There is clear synergy between the two.

You—the high-touch resource—are still far more valuable, we believe, than all the new and remarkable high-tech resources in today's health care. Your ability to touch the life of your patient, through your skillful listening, gentle probing, and steady encouragement, creates a therapeutic bond, which helps that patient feel significantly better—looked after and not just looked over. Within only a few private and very special moments, the patient's deepest fears and most intimate secrets can be divulged to you, as you draw on all of your skills, knowledge, and instincts to provide comfort. Surely, there is no communication more remarkable than this.

We hope this handbook of quick and easy-to-review communication techniques proves to be a ready reference over the years. We hope it offers effective solutions for the various situations you encounter, so that your overall communications with patients are as satisfying and fulfilling for you as they are helpful and therapeutic for your patients.

CME INFORMATION
AND TEST

Continuing Medical Education Credit

This program has been reviewed and is acceptable for up to 6 prescribed credit hours by the American Academy of Family Physicians. Term of approval is for one year from beginning distribution date of October 1, 2000, with option to request yearly approval.

Objectives

In writing this book, the authors' objectives are to

1. Help physicians improve their communication skills
2. Make practice more rewarding for physicians
3. Help physicians understand patients better
4. Decrease medicolegal risks to physicians

Disclosure

Author Joanne Desmond is president of Desmond Medical Communications (DMC) in Chicago. Some of the book's cases have been adapted from DMC's research.

Author Lanny Copeland, M.D., served from 1994 to 2000 as a member of the board of directors of the American Academy of Family Physicians (AAFP). He served as president of the AAFP in 1998–99 and has served as chair of its board of directors.

Instructions

1. Read the entire book, and answer all the questions on pages 240–244. Please indicate your answers by circling the letter that precedes each correct answer. (There is only one correct answer for each question. An answer key appears on pages 244–245.)

2. Print all required information on page 245.

   Carefully remove pages 240–245, and mail them to the sponsor of this activity: Jossey-Bass, Attention: CME Credit, 350 Sansome Street, San Francisco, CA 94104. (You may also photocopy the pages and return them to the sponsor.)

Questions

1. The average physician will conduct an average of how many interviews during his or her career?

   A 50,000

   B 90,000

   C 130,000

   D 240,000

2. Patient loyalty to a physician is best correlated with which of the following?

   A Good communication between patient and physician

   B Friendly office personnel

   C Health plans accepted by the physician

   D Proximity to a hospital

3. Women account for what percentage of consumer health care decisions?

   A 25 percent

   B 50 percent

   C 75 percent

   D 95 percent

4. Which of the following statements is true in regard to addressing patients?

   A All women should be addressed as "Ms."

   B All patients should be addressed by their first name.

   C All clergymen should be addressed as "Reverend."

   D Patients should be queried as to how they would like to be addressed.

5. Which of the following is not a trait of an Analytical patient?

   A Slow, soft voice

   B Few body gestures

   C Easily angered

   D Slow and logical responses

6. Which of the following is not a trait of an Amiable patient?

   A Very few facial expressions

   B May cry under stress

   C Considers family and friends very important

   D May become dependent on the physician

7. Which of the following is not a trait of an Expressive patient?

   A Likes variety and creativity

   B Oriented to the future

   C Enjoys being the center of attention

   D Slow and direct speech

8. Which body gesture is recommended when talking to a patient?

   A Leaning slightly forward and toward the patient

   B Standing up while taking the patient's history

   C Keeping arms folded

   D Constantly studying the patient's chart

9. In which of the following situations would a smile be inappropriate?

   A   As you walk into the room and greet the patient

   B   As you leave the room after a routine visit

   C   When the patient or family member has shared good news with you

   D   After telling the patient unexpected news

10. Which famous physician made the statement, "Listen to the patient; he is telling you the diagnosis"?

   A   Sir William Osler

   B   Jonas Salk, M.D.

   C   Walter Reed, M.D.

   D   Bob Graham, M.D.

11. Which part of a patient-physician encounter most often leads to the diagnosis?

   A   History

   B   Physical examination

   C   Laboratory data

   D   Radiographic studies

12. Studies show that physicians interrupt patients after what amount of time?

   A   7 seconds

   B   18 seconds

   C   45 seconds

   D   The time it takes for the patient to give a complete history

13. The skill of listening to a patient results in all of the following except which one?

   A   A stronger bond between patient and physician

   B   More satisfaction for the caregiver

CME Information and Test

C Decreased risk of malpractice

D Less time to make the diagnosis

14. When conducting patient interviews, all but which one of the following may be helpful?

A Open-ended questions

B Pausing

C Closed-ended questions

D Standing during the interview

15. A dissatisfied patient will share the fact of his or her dissatisfaction with how many others?

A 0

B 5

C 10

D 25

16. Which of the following is the original meaning of the word *doctor*, from Latin?

A Healer

B Teacher

C Stonecutter

D Pupil

17. Which of the following is not appropriate when explaining information to a patient?

A Drawing simple pictures to explain anatomy

B Using jargon that the patient will understand

C Only giving the patient a handout

D Asking the patient to repeat what was just said

18. Which of the following is not helpful in dealing with a patient's family?

A Greeting family members at each visit

B Giving family members a task that is helpful to the patient

C Identifying the key person

D Speaking to only one individual, who can in turn relay information to the other family members

19. In dealing with patients who speak a different language than the caregiver, which of the following is inappropriate?

A Asking one of the patient's young children to interpret

B Having an adult interpreter in the room and asking the patient to allow the interpreter to translate

C Drawing simple diagrams

D Making certain that medication instructions are written in the language the patient understands

20. In regard to wearing a white coat in the office, which of the following is incorrect?

A In general, it results in patients feeling more positive toward their physician.

B It makes an excellent first impression.

C It should not be worn when seeing children.

D It should always be clean and neat.

Answer Key

1. C

2. A

3. C

4. D

5. C

6. A

7. D

8. A

9. D

10. A

11. A

12. B

13. D

14. D

15. C

16. B

17. C

18. D

19. A

20. C

Instructions for Return of Answers to Sponsor

Please fill in your name and address below and return the answered questions to the sponsor of this activity, whose address appears in the instructions. You must return the answers by October 1, 2001. Your participation will be acknowledged within eight weeks by the sponsor.

_____

Name

_____

Complete Street Address

_____

_____

City/State/Zip

BIBLIOGRAPHY AND REFERENCES

Aburdene, P., and Naisbitt, J. *Megatrends for Women.* New York: Fawcett Columbine, 1992.

American Medical Association [brochure].

Baker, S. K. *Managing Patient Expectations.* San Francisco: Jossey-Bass, 1998.

Becker, M. H. "Patient Adherence to Prescribed Therapies." *Medical Care,* 1985, *23*(5), 539–555.

Beckman, H. B., and Frankel, R. M. "The Effect of Physician Behavior on the Collection of Data." *Annals of Internal Medicine,* 1984, *101*(5), 692–696.

Beckman, H. B., Markakis, K. M., Suchman, A. L., and Frankel, R. M. "The Doctor-Patient Relationship and Malpractice." *Archives of Internal Medicine,* 1994, *154,* 1365–1370.

Bell, C. S. "Difficult Patients Are Easy If You Know These Techniques." *Medical Economics,* Apr. 10, 1995, pp. 46–55.

Benson, H. *The Relaxation Response.* New York: Avon, 1975.

Berg, M. "Patient Education and the Physician-Patient Relationship." *Journal of Family Practice,* 1987, *24*(2), 169–172.

Bertakis, K. D., Roter, D., and Putnam, S. M. "The Relationship of Physician Medical Interview Style to Patient Satisfaction." *Journal of Family Practice,* 1991, *32(2),* 175–181.

Billings, J. A., and Stoeckle, J. D. *The Clinical Encounter.* Chicago: Yearbook Medical Publishers, 1989.

Braddock, C. H., III, and others. "Informed Decision Making in Outpatient Practice." *Journal of the American Medical Association,* 1999, *282*(24), 2313–2320.

Burack, R. C., and Carpenter, R. R. "The Predictive Value of the Presenting Complaint." *Journal of Family Practice,* 1983, *16*(4), 749–754.

Campbell, P. *Population Projections for States by Age, Sex, Race and Hispanic Origin: 1995–2025.* U.S. Census Bureau, Population Division, P25-1131. Washington, D.C.: U.S. Government Printing Office, May 1997.

Carr, A. C., and Ghosh, A. "Response of Phobic Patients to Direct Computer Assessment." *British Journal of Psychiatry,* 1983, *142,* 60–65.

Carter, W. B., Inui, T. S., Kukull, W. A., and Haigh, V. H. "Outcome-Based Doctor-Patient Interaction Analysis: II. Identifying Effective Provider and Patient Behavior." *Medical Care*, 1982, *20*(6), 550–566.

Cassell, E. *Talking with Patients.* Vol. 1: *The Theory of Doctor-Patient Communication.* Cambridge, Mass.: MIT Press, 1985.

DeFleur, M. H., and Desmond, J. "Physicians and Their 'Difficult' Patients." Forthcoming.

Delbanco, T. L. "Enriching the Doctor-Patient Relationship by Inviting the Patient's Perspective." *Annals of Internal Medicine,* 1992, *116*(5), 414–418.

Desmond, J. "Communicating with Multicultural Patients." *Life in Medicine,* Sept. 1994, pp. 7–25.

Desmond, J. "Communications: Patients' Yardstick for Quality." *The Digest: A Medical Liability and Risk Management Newsletter of St. Paul Fire & Marine Insurance Co. for Its Medical Liability Insurance Policyholders,* Fall 1990, pp. 1–3.

Desmond, J. "Effective Communications in Today's Managed Care." *Managed Care Medicine,* 1995, *2*(6), 14–18.

DiMatteo, M. R. "The Physician-Patient Relationship: Effects on the Quality of Health Care." *Clinical Obstetrics and Gynecology,* 1994, *37*(1), 149–161.

DiMatteo, M. R., Hays, R. D., and Prince, L. M. "Relationship of Physicians' Nonverbal Communication Skill to Patient Satisfaction, Appointment Noncompliance, and Physician Workload." *Health Psychology,* 1986, *5*(6), 581–594.

DiMatteo, M. R., Taranto, A., Friedman, H. S., and Prince, B. A. "Predicting Patient Satisfaction from Physicians' Nonverbal Communication Skills." *Medical Care,* 1980, *18*(4), 376–387.

Dowds, B. N., and Bibace, R. "Entry into the Health Care System: The Family's Decision-Making Process." *Family Medicine,* 1996, *28*(2), 114–118.

Dunn, J. J., and others. "Patient and House Officer Attitudes on Physician Attire and Etiquette." *Journal of the American Medical Association,* 1987, *257*(1), 65–68.

Ely, J. W., and others. "Perceived Causes of Family Physicians' Errors." *Journal of Family Practice,* 1995, *40*(4), 337–344.

Emerson, R. W. "Essays of Emerson." *Conduct of Life: Behavior.* Garden City, N.Y.: Garden City Publishing, 1941.

Engstrom, S., and Madlon-Kay, D. J. "Choosing a Family Physician: What Do Patients Want to Know?" *Minnesota Medicine,* 1998, *81,* 22–26.

Food and Drug Administration. "FDA National Consumer Surveys." Washington, D.C.: Food and Drug Administration, 1998, data released June 1999.

Gerteis, M., and others. "What Patients Really Want." *Health Management Quarterly,* 1993, *15*(3), 2–6.

Gibbs, N. "Sick and Tired." *Time,* July 31, 1989, p. 50.

Gillette, R. D., Filak, A., and Thorne, C. "First Name or Last Name: Which Do Patients Prefer?" *Journal of the American Board of Family Practice,* 1992, *5*(5), 517–522.

248

Gonzalez Del Rey, J. A., and Paul, R. I. "Preferences of Parents for Pediatric Emergency Physicians' Attire." *Pediatric Emergency Care*, 1995, *11*(6), 361–364.

Goodman, J. "Membership Services as a Revenue Center: Cost Justification and Marketing Impact of an Aggressive Service Program." Washington, D.C.: Technical Assistance Research Programs, 1999.

Gordon, G. H., Baker, L., and Levinson, W. "Physician-Patient Communication in Managed Care." *Western Journal of Medicine*, 1995, *163*(6), 527–531.

Grüninger, U. J. "Patient Education: An Example of One-to-One Communication." *Journal of Human Hypertension*, 1995, *9*(1), 15–25.

Gruppen, L. D., Wooliscroft J. O., and Wolf F. M. "The Contributions of Different Components of the Clinical Encounter in Generating and Eliminating Diagnostic Hypotheses." *Proceedings of the 27th Annual Conference on Research in Medical Education*, 1988, *27*, 242–247.

Hall, J. A., Roter, D. L., and Katz, N. R. "Meta-Analysis of Correlates of Provider Behavior in Medical Encounters." *Medical Care*, 1988, *26*(7), 657–672.

Jones, W.H.S. *Hippocrates*. Vol. 2. Cambridge, Mass.: Harvard University Press, 1923.

Kaplan, S. H., Greenfield, S., and Ware, J. E., Jr. "Assessing the Effects of Physician-Patient Interactions on the Outcomes of Chronic Disease." [Supplement.] *Medical Care*, 1989, *27*(3), S110–S127.

Kessler, R. C., and others. "Lifetime and 12-Month Prevalence of DSM-III-R Psychiatric Disorders in the United States." *Archives of General Psychiatry*, 1994, *51*, 12.

Korsch, B. M., Gozzi, E. K., and Francis, V. "Gaps in Doctor-Patient Communication: I. Doctor-Patient Interaction and Patient Satisfaction." *Pediatrics*, 1968, *42*(5), 855–871.

Korsch, B. M., and Negrete, V. F. "Doctor-Patient Communication." *Scientific American*, 1972, *227*(2), 66–74.

Langewitz, W. A., Eich, P., Kiss, A., and Wössmer, B. "Improving Communication Skills: A Randomized Controlled Behaviorally Oriented Intervention Study for Residents in Internal Medicine." *Psychosomatic Medicine*, 1998, *60*, 268–276.

Larsen, K. M., and Smith, C. K. "Assessment of Nonverbal Communication in the Patient-Physician Interview." *Journal of Family Practice*, 1981, *12*(3), 481–488.

Lester, G. W., and Smith, S. G. "Listening and Talking to Patients: A Remedy for Malpractice Suits?" *Western Journal of Medicine*, 1993, *158*(3), 268–272.

Levine, D. M. "Communicating with Chronic Disease Patients." *Comment: A Newsletter from the Miles Council for Physician-Patient Communication*, 1989, *3*(3), 1.

Levinson, W. "Physician-Patient Communication: A Key to Malpractice Prevention." *Journal of the American Medical Association*, 1994, *272*(20), 1619–1620.

Levinson, W. "Doctor-Patient Communication and Medical Malpractice: Implications for Pediatricians." *Pediatric Annals*, 1997, *26*(3), 186–193.

Levinson, W., and Roter, D. "The Effects of Two Continuing Medical Education Programs on Communication Skills of Practicing Primary Care Physicians." *Journal of General Internal Medicine,* 1993, *8,* 318–324.

Levinson, W., and Roter, D. "Physicians' Psychosocial Beliefs Correlate with Their Patient Communication Skills." *Journal of General Internal Medicine,* 1995, *10*(7), 375–379.

Levinson, W., Stiles, W. B., Inui, T. S., and Engle, R. "Physician Frustration in Communicating with Patients." *Medical Care,* 1993, *31*(4), 285–295.

Levinson, W., and others. "Physician-Patient Communication: The Relationship with Malpractice Claims Among Primary Care Physicians and Surgeons." *Journal of the American Medical Association,* 1997, *227*(7), 553–559.

Ley, P., Bradshaw, P. W., and Eaves, D. "A Method for Increasing Patients' Recall of Information Presented by Doctors." *Psychological Medicine,* 1973, *3,* 217–219.

Loverde, J. *The Complete Eldercare Planner: Where to Start, Which Questions to Ask, and How to Find Help.* (2nd ed.) New York: Times Books, 2000.

Luallin, M. D., and Sullivan, K. W. "The Patient's Advocate: A Six-Part Strategy for Building Market Share." *Group Practice Journal,* July/Aug. 1998, pp. 13–16.

Luecke, R. W., Rosselli, V. R., and Moss, J. M. "Economic Ramifications of 'Client' Dissatisfaction." *Group Practice Journal,* May 1991, pp. 8–18.

Mabeck, C. E., and Olesen, F. "Metaphorically Transmitted Diseases: How Do Patients Embody Medical Explanations?" *Group Practice Journal,* 1997, *14*(4), 271–278.

Marino, R. V., Rosenfeld, W., Narula, P., and Karakurum, M. "Impact of Pediatricians' Attire on Children and Parents." *Journal of Developmental and Behavioral Pediatrics,* 1991, *12*(2), 98–101.

Matsui, D., Cho, M., and Rieder, M. J. "Physicians' Attire as Perceived by Young Children and Their Parents: The Myth of the White Coat Syndrome." *Pediatric Emergency Care,* 1998, *14*(3), 198–201.

Mazzuca, S. A. "Does Patient Education in Chronic Disease Have Therapeutic Value?" *Journal of Chronic Diseases,* 1982, *35*(7), 521–529.

McAuliffe, K. "Computer Shrinks." *Self,* July 1991, pp. 103–104.

McKinstry, B., and Wang, J. "Putting on the Style: What Patients Think of the Way Their Doctor Dresses." *British Journal of General Practice,* 1991, *41,* 275–278.

Mehrabian, A. *Non-Verbal Communication.* Chicago: Aldine, 1972.

Myers, I., and Briggs, K. C. *Myers-Briggs Type Indicator.* Palo Alto, Calif.: Consulting Psychologists Press, 1990.

National Center for Health Statistics. *National Ambulatory Medical Care Survey.* Advance Data no. 305, May 20, 1999.

National Council on Patient Information and Education. "Educate Before You Medicate: Talk About Prescriptions." [http://www.talkaboutrx.org]. 2000.

Nichols, L. O., and Mirvis, D. M. "Physician-Patient Communication: Does It Matter?" *Tennessee Medicine*, Mar. 1998, pp. 94–96.

Osler, W. "Lecture to Medical Students." *Albany Medical Annals*, 1899, *20*, 307.

Peterson, M. C., and others. "Contributions of the History, Physical Examination, and Laboratory Investigation in Making Medical Diagnoses." *Western Journal of Medicine*, Feb. 1992, pp. 163–165.

Realini, T., Kalet, A., and Sparling, J. "Interruption in the Medical Interaction." *Archives of Family Medicine*, 1995, *4*, 1028–1033.

Reid, R. H., and Merrill, D. W. *Personal Styles and Effective Performance*. Radnor, Pa.: Chilton, 1981.

Rosenberg, E. E., Lussier, M.-T., and Beaudoin, C. "Lessons for Clinicians from Physician-Patient Communication Literature." *Archives of Family Medicine*, 1997, *6*, 279–283.

Roter, D. L., and Hall, J. A. *Doctors Talking with Patients/Patients Talking with Doctors: Improving Communication in Medical Visits*. Westport, Conn.: Auburn House, 1992.

Roter, D. L., and Hall, J. A. "Strategies for Enhancing Patient Adherence to Medical Recommendations." *Journal of the American Medical Association*, 1994, *272*(1), 80.

Roter, D. L., and others. "Communication Patterns of Primary Care Physicians." *Journal of the American Medical Association*, 1997, *277*(4), 350–356.

Rouwenhorst, R. C. "In Your Defense: The Physician's Role in the Defense of Medical Liability Claims." *The Digest, A Medical Liability and Risk Management Newsletter*, 1996, *24*(3), 1–5.

Ruhl, T. "Use Analogies to Help Patients Understand Medical Concepts." *FP Report: American Academy of Family Physicians*. [http://www.aafp.org/fpr/]. July 1999.

Rundle, A. K., Carvalho, M., and Robinson, M. (eds.). *Honoring Patient Preferences: A Guide to Complying with Multicultural Patient Requirements*. San Francisco: Jossey-Bass, 1999.

Sanders, P. S., and McBride, D. L. "Malpractice Prevention: Good Doctor-Patient Communication." *Minnesota Medicine*, Feb. 1998, pp. 27–30.

Schmidley, A. D., and Gibson, C. *Profile of the Foreign-Born Population in the United States: 1997*. U.S. Census Bureau, Current Population Reports, Series P23-195. Washington, D.C.: U.S. Government Printing Office, 1999.

Shortell, S. M., and others. "The Performance of Intensive Care Units: Does Good Management Make a Difference?" *Medical Care*, 1994, *32*(5) 508–525.

Slomski, A. "Will Patients Leave You for Cheaper Care?" *Medical Economics*, Aug. 21, 1995, pp. 47–57.

Stevens, S. "Better Communication Skills Seen Key to Improving Bedside Manner." *Physicians Financial News*, 1992, *10*(2), 1.

Stewart, D. W., and others. "Information Search and Decision Making in the Selection of Family Health Care." *Journal of Health Care Marketing*, 1989, *9*(2), 29–39.

Stewart, M. A. "Effective Physician-Patient Communication and Health Outcomes: A Review." *Canadian Medical Association Journal*, 1995, *152*(9), 1423–1433.

Stewart, M. A., and Roter, D. L. (eds.). *Communicating with Medical Patients.* Thousand Oaks, Calif.: Sage, 1989.

Street, R. L., Jr. "Communicative Styles and Adaptations in Physician-Parent Consultations." *Social Science and Medicine*, 1992, *34*(10), 1155–1163.

Street, R. L., Jr., and Wiemann, J. M. "Differences in How Physicians and Patients Perceive Physicians' Relational Communication." *Southern Speech Communication Journal*, Summer 1988, pp. 420–440.

Suchman, A. L., Markakis, K., Beckman, H. B., and Frankel, R. "A Model of Empathic Communication in the Medical Interview." *Journal of the American Medical Association*, 1997, *227*(8), 678–682.

Tannen, D. *That's Not What I Meant!* New York: Ballantine, 1986.

van Dulmen, A. M., Verhaak, P.F.M., and Bilo, H.J.G. "Shifts in Doctor-Patient Communication During a Series of Outpatient Consultations in Non-Insulin-Dependent Diabetes Mellitus." *Patient Education and Counseling*, 1997, *30*, 227–237.

Ver Berkmoes, R. "Physician Fashion: It Pays to Dress Well." *American Medical News*, 1988, *31*(19), 27–30.

Weber, D. "Convenience: You Still Have a Way to Go." (Patient attitude survey.) *Medical Economics*, Aug. 21, 1995, pp. 68–79.

White, J., Levinson, W., and Roter, D. "Oh, by the Way . . . : The Closing Moments of the Medical Visit." *Journal of General Internal Medicine*, 1994, *9*, 24–28.

Wolf, F. M., Wooliscroft, J. O., Calhoun, J. G., and Boxar, G. J. "A Controlled Experiment in Teaching Students to Respond to Patients' Emotional Concerns." *Journal of Medical Education*, 1987, *62*, 25–34.

Young, F. "Questions About Your Medicine? Then Go Ahead—Ask." *FDA Consumer*, Oct. 1987, pp. 2–3.

RECOMMENDED READING

These works are listed alphabetically by title.

The Clinical Encounter, by J. Andrew Billings and John D. Stoeckle. Chicago: Yearbook Medical Publishers, 1989.

Communicating with Medical Patients, edited by Moira Stewart and Debra Roter. Thousand Oaks, Calif.: Sage, 1989.

Communicating with Patients: Improving Communication, Satisfaction, and Compliance, by Philip Ley. London: Croom Helm, 1988.

The Complete Eldercare Planner: Where to Start, Which Questions to Ask, and How to Find Help, by Joy Loverde. (3rd ed.). New York: Times Books, 2000.

Conversation Failure: Case Studies in Doctor-Patient Communication, by Frederic W. Platt. Tacoma, Wash.: Life Sciences Press, 1992.

"Difficult Patients Are Easy If You Know These Techniques," by C. S. Bell. *Medical Economics,* Apr. 10, 1995, pp. 46–55.

Doctors Talking with Patients/Patients Talking with Doctors: Improving Communication in Medical Visits, by Debra L. Roter and Judith A. Hall. Westport, Conn.: Auburn House, 1992.

Managing Patient Expectations: The Art of Finding and Keeping Loyal Patients, by Susan Keane Baker. San Francisco: Jossey-Bass, 1998.

Monograph on Patient Satisfaction, Practice Pointers: A Practice Management Guide for the Osteopathic Physician. Chicago: American Osteopathic Association, 1996.

Personal Styles and Effective Performance, by R. H. Reid and D. W. Merrill. Radnor, Pa.: Chilton, 1981.

Talking with Patients: A Basic Clinical Skill, by Philip R. Myerscough. (2nd ed.). Oxford: Oxford University Press, 1992.

Talking with Patients. Vol. 1: *The Theory of Doctor-Patient Communication,* by Eric J. Cassell. Cambridge, Mass.: MIT Press, 1985.

Talking with Patients. Vol. 2: *Clinical Technique,* by Eric J. Cassell. Cambridge, Mass.: MIT Press, 1985.

INDEX

A

Abrazzo, 214
Aburdene, P., 16
Accessories, worn by clinicians, 227–229
Active listening, 96–99; body language for, 97, 98; goal of, 96; on telephone, 99; vocal confirmation in, 98
Adherence: communication as increasing, 5; techniques for encouraging, to medications, 170–179. *See also* Explanations
Agency for Health Policy, 17
Alternative remedies, medications' interactions with, 177–178
American College of Physician Executives, 78
American Health Lawyers Association, 8
Americans, use of term, 206
Amiable patients, 55–60, 133, 163; getting on track with, 58; identifying, 56; preferences of, 39, 55; relationships of, 56; under stress, 56–57; time orientation of, 55; working with, 58–60
Analogies, used in patient education, 141–143
Analytical patients, 47–54; getting on track with, 49–50; identifying, 48–49; preferences of, 39, 47; under stress, 49; time orientation of, 47–48; working with, 50–55
Apparel, clinician, 221–226

B

Baker, L., 4
Baker, S. K., 231
Beaudoin, C., 2
Becker, M. H., 5
Beckman, H. B., 7, 102–103, 126
Bell, C. S., 223
Benson, H., 20
Bertakis, K. D., 5, 112, 130
Billings, J. A., 130, 184–185
Bilo, H.J.G., 3, 104, 131
Body language, 71–94; as aid in determining family leader, 193–194; for communicating to family members, 190, 198–199; examples of negative, 71, 72; eye contact, 30, 85–88, 98, 131, 149, 190, 215–216; facial expressions, 28, 30–31, 84–85, 97; general tips on, 91, 93; gestures, 76–80, 215; for giving explanations, 149; handshakes, 26, 28–29, 35, 213–214; head movements, 88–90; importance of, 72–74; for listening, 80–82, 131–134; with multicultural patients, 213–216; patient perceptions of, 74, 75–76, 92; positive, 92; for positive first impressions, 28–32; putting down colleagues, 90–91; shoulder orientation, 30, 82–83, 97, 190; to signal who talks when, 198–199; sitting positions, 80–84, 149
Boxar, G. J., 10

Braddock, C. H., 136–137
Bradshaw, P. W., 184
Briggs, K. C., 41
Brigham and Women's Hospital (Boston), 222
Burack, R. C., 129

C

Calhoun, J. G., 10
Campbell, P., 204
Carpenter, R. R., 129
Carr, T., 73
Carter, W. B., 138
Carvalho, M., 219
Charts: avoiding focusing on, 31–32; information brought in by patient on, 54; name pronunciations on, 25–26; small-talk topics on, 33–34
Cho, M., 223, 230
Clinical Encounter, The (Billings and Stoeckle), 130
Clinicians: introductions, 27–28; patient perceptions of body language of, 74, 75–76, 92; professional satisfaction of, xiv, 4, 238; social styles of, 66–69; speaking in foreign languages, 205–206; who can benefit from this book, xvi. *See also* Physicians; Professional image
Closed-ended questions, 115–122; advantages of, 115–116; announcing series of, 117; avoiding "right answer questions," 118; disadvantages of, 117; patients preferring, 119–120; phrasing for, 116–117, 118; rephrased as open-ended, 120–122; when to use, 118–119
Closings: for appointments, 34–36; for explanations, 163; reflective listening in, 101
Clothing, clinician, 221–226
Coining, 217
Communication: benefits of using specific techniques for, 11; delegation of, 10; as essential clinical skill, 10; importance of body language in, 72–74; meaning

of term, 138; social styles as affecting, 40–41, 67–69; as unique element of medicine, 237–238
Communication skills: benefits of, 1–9; as capable of being learned, 9–10
Community resources: for Analytical patients, 52; for family, 195–196
Complaints: filed by family members, 200; time and cost of handling, 3; as valuable feedback, 15
Compliance: communication as increasing, 5; techniques for encouraging, with medications, 170–179. *See also* Explanations
Conrad, H., 238
Continuing medical education (CME): information, 239; test, 240–245
Copeland, L. R., 21
Cost: of acquiring new versus keeping current patients, 13; adjusting, when physician late for appointment, 44, 66; of handling complaints, 3; of lost patient, 14–15; of medications, 172–173
Cousins, N., 34
Crying patients, 56–57, 107–108
Cultural issues. *See* Multicultural patients
Culturegrams, 219
Cupping, 216–217
Curanderas, 213

D

Decision making: health care, by women, 16; shared with patients, 136–137
DeFleur, M. H., 137, 187
Delbanco, T. L., 189
Denham, C., 201
Depression, listening for emotional clues of, 127–129
Desmond, J., 19, 36, 137, 187
Diagnoses: accuracy of, and communication skills, 2; explaining tests for, 142–143; listening's role in, 2, 95; of psychosocial disorders, 129
diCosola, R., 238
DiMatteo, M. R., 4, 5, 10, 74, 166

Doctor, original meaning of, 135. *See also* Physicians

"Doctors' House Call," 16, 151, 152

Drawings, for patient education, 147–148, 207

Driving patients, 42–47, 133; getting on track with, 44–45; identifying, 43; preferences of, 39, 42; relationships of, 43; under stress, 44; time orientation of, 42; working with, 45–46

Dunn, J. J., 24, 222

E

Eaves, D., 184

Ely, J. W., 20, 89

Emerson, R. W., 73

Emotions: depression as revealed in, 127–129; empathic listening and, 104–108; inappropriate but well-meaning responses to, 108–110; listening for clues related to, 123–134; open-ended questions to reveal problems with, 130–131; questions arousing, 171–172; sharing, with patient's family, 191; talking with patients about, 44, 58, 65–66, 87–88. *See also* Empathic listening

Empathic listening, 96, 104–108; as bonding agent, 105; examples of verbal responses/cues for, 104, 107; goal of, 96; opportunities missed for, 105–107; with weeping patients, 107–108

Engle, R., 188

English-as-a-second-language patients. *See* Multicultural patients

Engstrom, S., 17

Expectations, patient, 163–164, 222

Explanations: advantages of giving clear, 136, 138–139; body language for giving, 149; closing for, 163; as contributing to patient satisfaction, 138; feedback from patients on, 163–164; to get results, 135–138; handouts for, 146–147; maps accompanying, 159; for multicultural patients, 144, 208–209;

to reduce risk of malpractice lawsuits, 136; techniques for, about medications, 168–170; time saved with clear, 139; time spent giving, 136; verbal techniques for, 140–145; visual aids for, 64, 147–149, 207; vocabulary for, 150–163; why patients misunderstand, 137–138

Expressive patients, 60–66, 133; getting on track with, 62; identifying, 61; preferences of, 39, 60; relationships of, 60–61; under stress, 61–62; time orientation of, 60; working with, 62–66

Eye contact, 85–88; in active listening, 98; in first appointment, 30; focal points for maintaining, 30; for giving explanations, 149; glasses and, 87–88, 131–132, 228; for listening for emotional clues, 131; with multicultural patients, 215–216; when communicating to family members, 190

F

Facial expressions, 84–85; for active listening, 97; in first appointment, 30–31; smiling, 28, 84

Family members, 187–201; as advocates for patients, 188; angry, 58–59, 199–200; asking for support from, 189, 194–195; avoiding ignoring, 200–201; dealing with difficult, 196–201; family's main contact person, 192–194; giving tasks to, 190, 206; greeting, 26, 27, 190; as helpful with bad news, 196; of multicultural patients, 190, 206, 211–213; as problem for clinicians, 187–188; recommending community resources to, 195–196; speaking for patient, 188, 196–199; telephone communication with, 194, 195; tips for communicating with, 189–192

Feedback: on body language, 93; lack of, from patients, 15, 163; on patient understanding of medications, 185–186; on patient's service expectations, 163–164. *See also* Reflective listening

Feelings. *See* Emotions
Figures of speech, used in patient education, 143
Filak, A., 24
First impressions, 14–15; based on clinician's appearance, 221; body language for positive, 28–32
Folk remedies: medications' interactions with, 177–178; among multicultural patients, 216–219
Food and Drug Administration (FDA), 165, 166–167
Foreign languages, clinicians' use of, 205–206
Francis, V., 9, 130, 155, 156
Frankel, R., 7, 102–103, 126
Frowning, 84–85

G

Garvey, M., 8
Gestures, 76–80, 215
Gibson, C., 204
Gillette, R. D., 24
Glasses, 87–88, 131–132, 228
Goodman, J., 15, 16
Gordon, G. H., 4
Gosfield, A., 8
Gozzi, E. K., 9, 130, 155, 156
Greenfield, S., 6, 111, 138
Grooming, clinician, 229–232
Group Practice Journal, 13
Grüninger, U. J., 5, 136
Gruppen, L. D., 95

H

Haigh, V. H., 138
Hairstyles, clinician, 229–230
Hall, J. A., 6, 19, 138, 139, 171
Handouts, used for patient education, 146–147
Handshakes, 26, 28–29, 35, 213–214
Hays, R. D., 4, 74
Head movements, 88–91
"Hey, you" pronouns, 25
Hippocrates, 222

History: diagnostic role of, 95; receiving versus taking, 112
Honoring Patient Preferences (Rundle, Carvalho, and Robinson), 219
Houfek, A., 223
Humor, 34, 61

I

Immigration, 204
Information: avoiding overload of, 151, 169; brought in by patients, 53–55; desired by family members, 188; essential, when explaining medications to patients, 167, 179–183
Instructions: maps accompanying, 51, 159; about medications, 165, 166–167, 183–185, 208
Interpreters, with multicultural patients, 209–210, 211–212
Introductions, using patient names in, 27–28
Inui, T. S., 138, 188

J

Jargon, 151–159; common medical terminology as, 152–153, 155–156; effect of, on patients, 153–154; exercise on reducing, 158–159; tips on using, 154–155; used by patients, 102, 156–157; written versus spoken, 157–158. *See also* Vocabulary
Jewelry, 227–228
Jones, W.H.S., 222

K

Kagawa Singer, M., 204
Kaiser Family Foundation, 17
Kalet, A., 111
Kaplan, S. H., 6, 111, 138
Karakurum, M., 223
Katz, N. R., 6, 19, 138
Kessler, R. C., 129
Koop, C. E., 230

Korsch, B. M., 9, 130, 155, 156
Kukull, W. A., 138

L

Larsen, K. M., 80, 81, 89
Laughter, 34, 62
Lawsuits. *See* Malpractice lawsuits
Lester, G. W., 7–8
Levine, D. M., 189
Levinson, W., 4, 7, 10, 136, 139, 185, 188
Ley, P., 184
Listening, 95–134; active, 96–99; body language for, 80–82, 131–134; closed-ended questions employed in, 115–122; diagnostic role of, 2, 95; for emotional clues, 123–134; empathic, 96, 104–108; inappropriate but well-meaning responses when, 108–110; open-ended questions employed in, 110–115; prompters used in, 122–123; reasons for patients' lack of, 138; reflective, 96, 99–104; on telephone, 99
Loverde, J., 191
Luallin, M. D., 13, 16, 17
Luecke, R. W., 13, 14–15
Lussier, M.-T., 2

M

Mabeck, C. E., 144
Madlon-Kay, D. J., 17
Mal de ojo (evil eye), 216
Malpractice lawsuits: communication as reducing risk of, 7–8, 136; reasons for, 7–8, 17
Managing Patient Expectations (Baker), 231
Maps, accompanying referrals or orders for tests, 51, 159
Marino, R. V., 223
Markakis, K., 7, 126
Matsui, D., 223, 230
Mazzuca, S. A., 138
McAuliffe, K., 73
McBride, D. L., 8
McKinstry, B., 222, 223, 228

Media: encouraging patients to take active health care role, xiii; medication reports in, 175
Medical Economics, 4, 16–17, 18, 223
Medical practice: communication as unique element of, 237–238; core competencies necessary for, 8
Medications, 165–186; aids for making, easy to take, 178–179; checking for patient understanding of, 185–186; checkups on, 178; essential information to give patients about, 167, 179–183; examples of miscommunication with patients about, 165, 203; financial hurdles to patients' taking, 172–173; folk or alternative remedies and, 177–178; frequency of prescribing, 166; instructions about, 165, 166–167, 183–185, 208; media reports on, 175; over-the-counter, 183; patient's attitudes and past experiences with, 175–176; requiring dosage adjustment, 174; side effects of, 174–175; techniques for avoiding patients' stopping, 170–179; techniques for explaining, 168–170
Megatrends for Women (Aburdene and Naisbitt), 16
Mehrabian, A., 72, 78, 82
Men: crying by, 108; preferred shoulder orientation of clinician with, 86, 97; touching multicultural patients, 214
Merrill, D. W., 38, 40
Metaphors: clinician use of, 143–145; patient use of, 144–145
Mirvis, D. M., 1
H. C. Moffett Hospital (San Francisco), 222
Moss, J. M., 13, 14–15
Multicultural patients, 203–219; body language with, 213–216; dealing with families of, 27, 190, 206, 211–213; defining, 204–205; establishing relationships with, 205–206; examples of miscommunication with, 165, 203, 209–210, 211; folk remedies of, 216–219; giving family members of, a task, 190, 206; immigrant background of, 204;

Multicultural patients, *continued*
overcoming language barriers with,
205–206, 207–214; preferring closed-
ended questions, 120; resources on, 219;
touching, 29, 213–214; using interpreters with, 209–210, 211–212; using
metaphors in explanations with, 144;
vocabulary used with, 206, 210–211
Myers, I., 41
Myers-Briggs Type Indicator (MBTI), 41

N

Naisbitt, J., 16
Name badges, clinician, 229
Names, patient: in introductions, 27–28;
pronouncing, 25–26; tips on using,
22–28, 62–64; updating, 26–27
Narula, P., 223
National Center for Health Statistics, 166
National Committee for Quality Assur-
ance (NCQA), 7
National Council on Patient Information
and Education, 167
National Health Lawyers Association, 8
"Negative," use of term, 155
New patients: body language with, 28–32;
closings for appointment with, 34–36;
communication techniques for use
with, 19–22; cost of acquiring, versus
keeping current patients, 13; first impressions with, 14–15; room layout
and, 32; small talk with, 32–34; using
patient names with, 22–28
Nichols, L. O., 1
Non-Verbal Communication (Mehrabian), 72
Nonverbal communication. *See* Body
language

O

Office, professional image in, 232–235
Olesen, F., 144
Open-ended questions: advantages of,
111; closed-ended questions rephrased
as, 120–122; at first appointment with
new patients, 21–22; about folk remedies, 217–219; for medication checkups, 178; pauses as, 123; phrasing for,

112–113, 113–115; to reveal emotional
problems, 130–131; timing of, 113
Osler, W., 95
Outcomes, communication as improving,
6
Over-the-counter medications, 183

P

Passivity, patient, 103–104, 153–154
Patient education. *See* Explanations
Patient satisfaction: clear explanations as
necessary for, 139; explanations as contributing to, 138; with improved communication, 4–5, 7
Patient turnover: xiii; cost of, 13, 14–15;
reasons for, 16–17
Patients: Amiable, 39, 55–60, 163; Analytical, 39, 47–55; dependent on physicians, 57; Driving, 39, 42–46, 133;
expectations of, 163–164, 222; Expressive, 39, 60–66, 133; factors affecting
physician choice by, 16–19; information brought in by, 53–55; loyalty/
retention of, 4; names of, 22–28, 62–
64; passivity of, 103–104, 153–154;
perceptions by, 7–8, 19, 37, 74, 75–76,
92; perks popular with, 18; priorities
of, 17–18; weeping, 107–108. *See also*
Multicultural patients; New patients
Paulson, T., 85
Pauses, 170, 207
Pediatrics: figures of speech used in, 143;
metaphors used in, 143–144; white
coats worn by clinicians in, 223
Perceptions: of clinicians' body language,
74, 75–76, 92; importance of, 19; personalities as affecting, 37; as reason for
filing lawsuits, 7–8, 17; as reason for
leaving physicians, 17
Peterson, M. C., 2, 95
Physical examinations, narrations during,
140–141
Physician Insurers Association of America, 8
Physicians: factors affecting patients'
choice of, 16–19; and original meaning
of "doctor," 135; patient dependence

on, 57; patient priorities in communication with, 17; reasons patients leave, 4, 16–17; self-assessment of communication skills, 9; time spent giving explanations, 136; on why patients misunderstand explanations, 137–138. *See also* Clinicians; Professional image
Pointing, 79
"Positive," use of term, 155
Prince, L. M., 4, 74
Professional image, 221–235; and accessories, 227–229; and apparel, 221–226; and grooming, 229–232; and office environment, 232–235; and telephone usage, 235; and weight and fitness, 226–227
Prompters, 122–123
Proxemics. *See* Social distance
Psychosocial disorders, missed diagnosis of, 129
Putnam, S. M., 5, 112, 130

Q

Quality of care, patients' rating of, and communication skills, 6–7
Questions: closed-ended, 115–122; to determine patient's likelihood of taking medications, 171; fewer, with clear explanations, 139; interrupting patients' stories, 102–104; with multicultural patients, 208, 209; open-ended, 21–22, 110–115, 130–131, 178, 217–219; "right answer," 118

R

Realini, T., 111
Recommendations, word-of-mouth, for choosing physicians, 16
Reflective listening, 96, 99–104; examples of, 100; goal of, 96; techniques for, 100–101; timing of, 102–103; using patient's vocabulary in, 102
Reid, R. H., 38, 40
Relationships: of Amiable patients, 56; of Analytical patients, 48; of Driving patients, 43; of Expressive patients, 60–61; social style information as useful for all, 41

"Remarkable/unremarkable," use of terms, 156
Rieder, M. J., 223, 230
Robinson, M., 219
Room layout, 32
Rosenberg, E. E., 2
Rosenfeld, W., 223
Rosselli, V. R., 13, 14–15
Roter, D., 3, 5, 6, 10, 19, 112, 130, 138, 139, 171, 185
Rouwenhorst, R. C., 147
Ruhl, T., 142
Rundle, A. K., 219

S

Sanders, P. S., 8
Satisfaction: clinicians' professional, xiv, 4, 238; patient, 4–5, 7, 138, 139
Schmidley, A. D., 204
Self-assessment, of physicians' communication skills, 9
Shoes, 228–229
Shortell, S. M., 6
Shoulder orientation: for active listening, 97; in first appointment, 30; gender and, 86, 97; in sitting position, 82–83; when communicating to family members, 190
Similes, used in patient education, 141–143
Sitting positions, 80–84, 149
Slomski, A., 4, 17
Small talk, 32–34, 35
Smiling, 28, 84
Smith, C. K., 80, 81
Smith, S. G., 7–8, 89
Social distance: with multicultural patients, 84, 213; between patient and clinician, 49–50, 83–84
Social styles, 38–42; of Amiable patients, 39, 55–60; of Analytical patients, 39, 47–55; broadening communication styles using, 67–69; of clinicians, 66–69; determining, 41–42, 43, 48–49, 56, 61; of difficult patients, 66–67; of Driving patients, 39, 42–47; of Expressive patients, 39, 60–66

Sparling, J., 111
Statistics: about medication side effects, 175; used in patient education, 145
"Steepling," 77–78
Stewart, M. A., 6
Stiles, W. B., 188
Stoeckle, J. D., 2, 130, 184–185
Street, R. L., Jr., 9
Stress, social styles of patients and, 44, 49, 56–57, 61–62
Suchman, A. L., 7, 126
Sullivan, K. W., 13, 16, 17

T

Tannen, D., 29, 102
Telephone: listening to patients on, 99; professional manner while using, 235; speaking with patient's family on, 194, 195
That's Not What I Meant (Tannen), 29
Thorne, C., 24
Ties, 227
Time: optimum, for open-ended questions, 113; required to handle complaints, 3; saved with clear explanations, 139, 186; saved with improved communication skills, 2–4; spent by physicians giving explanations, 136; waiting, compensating patients for, 44, 66
Time orientation: of Amiable patients, 55; of Analytical patients, 47–48; of Driving patients, 42; of Expressive patients, 60
Titles, using patients', 24–25, 62–64
Touching: at first appointments, 29; handshakes, 26, 28–29, 35, 213–214; multicultural patients, 29, 213–214
Training, in communication skills, 9–10

U

University of Texas, Southwestern Medical Center, Arthritis Educator Program, 150

V

van Dulmen, A. M., 3, 104, 131
Verhaak, P.F.M., 3, 104, 131
Visual aids: for patient education, 64, 147–149; used with multicultural patients, 207
Vocabulary: alarm words, 159–160; "Americans," 206; "but" versus "and," 162–163; for closed-ended questions, 116–117, 118; "hot buttons," 160–161; hurtful terms, 150–151; for medication explanations, 179–183; for open-ended questions, 112–113, 113–115; personalized, for explanations, 168; "positive" and "negative," 155; positive spin words, 162; "remarkable/unremarkable," 156; used by patient, 102, 144–145, 156–157; used with multicultural patients, 206, 210–211. *See also* Jargon

W

Waiting time: compensating patient for, 44, 66; staff checking on patients during, 234
Wallace, M., 123
Wang, J., 222, 223, 228
Ware, J. E., Jr., 6, 111, 138
Weber, D., 18
Weeping patients, 56–57, 107–108
White, J., 139, 185
Wiemann, J. M., 9
Wolf, F., 9, 10, 95
Women: avoiding familiar language with, 24–25; as health care decision makers, 16; as main contact person in family, 193; preferred shoulder orientation of clinician with, 86, 97; touching multicultural, 214
Wooliscroft, J. O., 10, 95
Writing pads, for patient education, 148

Y

Young, F., 180

ABOUT THE AUTHORS

Joanne Desmond is president of Desmond Medical Communications, with offices in Chicago and Boston. She has extensive experience as an award-winning science and medical reporter, television news anchor, medical talk-show host, communications consultant, and international keynote speaker.

Articles by or about her have been published in *Medical Economics*, the *Los Angeles Times, Physician Executive, Managed Care Medicine, Hospital Risk Management, Managed Healthcare News*, and other medical journals.

Desmond was a scholarship student at Northwestern University's School of Speech and Communication. Her graduate work was at the University of Missouri School of Journalism, where she won the school's annual Wilson Prize for Best Medical Writing. She also received a National Science Foundation Scholarship to the University of San Francisco.

As Boston's first TV news anchorwoman (and one of the first in the nation), she co-anchored both the noontime news and evening news for the city's CBS affiliate. She was also WBZ-TV's science and medical reporter. Her credits as a writer and producer include award-winning series for Public Television stations WGBH-TV (Boston), KLRN-TV (Austin, Texas), and the Armed Forces Network overseas. "Doctors' House Call," the prime-time medical information talk show that she hosted, won the national CableACE award, the "Emmy" of cable television.

Desmond and her staff of trainers conduct workshops and license trainers in patient communications and interstaff communications as well as in media and presentation skills for major health care associations and organizations throughout the nation and abroad. More than three thousand physicians and other health care professionals have attended Desmond Medical Communications workshops and other programs over the past two decades.

Lanny R. Copeland, M.D., is a family physician who practiced for eighteen years in the small town of Moultrie, Georgia. In 1994, he joined the faculty of the Southwest Georgia Family Practice Residency program in Albany and is currently vice president of primary care development for Phoebe Putney Health Systems, also in Albany, Georgia. He holds the rank of professor in the Department of Family and Community Medicine at Mercer School of Medicine in Macon, as well as clinical associate professor in the Department of Family Medicine at the Medical College of Georgia in Augusta. In 1985, he was recognized as the Family Medicine Educator of the Year and in 1988 as Family Physician of the Year by the Georgia Academy of Family Physicians. He served on the board of directors of the American Board of Family Practice from 1989 to 1994 and was its president in 1993–94.

From 1994 to the present, he has been a member of the board of directors of the American Academy of Family Physicians (AAFP). He is a past president of the AAFP and has served as chair of its board of directors.

ABOUT DESMOND MEDICAL COMMUNICATIONS

Desmond Medical Communications provides keynote addresses and workshops on numerous topics:

- Key communication skills for difficult patient encounters
- Successful interstaff communication in a time of change
- Saying no positively; giving denials that patients can accept
- Essential communication skills for today's nurses
- Presentation and media skills training
- The voice of authority; improving your vocal impact
- Telephone techniques for improved patient communication

For more information, or to schedule a workshop, contact DMC at 333 North Michigan Ave., Suite 934, Chicago, IL 60601; telephone (800) 942-4399; e-mail JDesmond33@aol.com; Web page www.Speakers.com/JDesmond.htm.

We appreciate hearing about any additional communication tips or techniques you have found useful in dealing with your patients. Please be sure to include your name and contact information so that if these tips or anecdotes are used in our future publications, credit can be appropriately given. Thank you.

Joanne Desmond
President
Desmond Medical Communications